The Strange Story of
FALSE TEETH

The Strange Story of
FALSE TEETH

John Woodforde

Foreword by James Laver

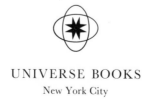

UNIVERSE BOOKS
New York City

*Published in the United States of America in 1970
by Universe Books
381 Park Avenue South
New York City, 10016*

© *John Woodforde 1968*

Library of Congress Catalog Card Number: 73-97597

SBN 87663-118-9

Printed in Great Britain

Contents

Acknowledgements

I am grateful to Mr. J. A. Donaldson, Curator of the British Dental Association's Museum and Editor of the *Dental Journal*, for reading the typescript and advising; to Miss E. Muriel Spencer, B.D.A. Librarian, and to the staff of the London Library for help with sources; to the Countess of Longford, Mr. H. Colin Davis and Sir Compton Mackenzie for suggestions; and to Colonel P. C. Mills for telling me about the charitable work of his Lascelles great-aunts in making artificial teeth for the indigent toothless.

May 1968   J.W.

Illustrations

Foreword

As the philosopher Keyserling once remarked: 'Whoever profoundly understands a superficial part of Life necessarily gains metaphysical insight along with it.' Perhaps Mr. Woodforde would hardly claim to be a metaphysician: he is certainly a social historian of no mean stature. If his subject may seem superficial at first glance he certainly gets down to the roots of it (it is astonishing how difficult it is to talk about it at all without using images derived from dentistry), and has thrown a flood of light on all kinds of other things.

Presumably primitive man had excellent teeth, or how could he have masticated raw flesh or gnawed the bones of bison? Cooking perhaps and the advent of agriculture may have set him on the wrong track. 'There ain't no bones in pudding', and a mess of pottage cannot have helped in the preservation of teeth. Tooth decay must have been well advanced by the time of the Neolithic culture; and from the Bronze Age we actually have evidence of it. It was found, Mr. Woodforde tells us, in seven skulls out of thirty-two dating from this period. And we must remember that, at that time, most people died at a comparatively early age. Toothache is as old as history.

Yet, almost at once (we learn for our comfort) men began to look for a remedy. The Etruscans 'excelled all at mechanical skill with dental appliances'. The Greeks and Romans did clever things with gold wire; and there was no attempt to conceal such contrivances. On the contrary they conferred a kind of social distinction, like the gold teeth of the inhabitants of Harlem a generation ago. Mr. Woodforde certainly makes a valid point when he tells us that 'vanity rather than the desire to chew better' was the dominant motive in the development of dentistry.

And indeed, why not? Good teeth have always been the mark of youth and vigour; bad teeth, or no teeth at all, the mark of age and decrepitude. Pleasure is expressed by showing one's teeth. Perhaps it is because the first pleasure was pleasure in devouring something that we still show our teeth when we smile; and if they are missing the effect is quite spoiled.

It is curious that the effect is even more completely spoiled if only one front tooth is missing. The young vandals who deface posters by adding moustaches to girls' faces sometimes also black out one of the teeth – and an attractive young woman is immediately transformed into a hag.

Mr. Woodforde's book should make us all thankful that we live in the age of modern dentistry. He gives innumerable examples of the miseries – physical and mental – endured by people of the past. In his old age the eloquent John Wilkes could hardly utter an intelligible word, and there must have been many with a similar disadvantage. Only Voltaire was witty enough to make a joke of it: 'Sir,' said Boswell, 'do you speak English?' and Voltaire replied, 'Sir, in order to speak English it is necessary to place the tongue between the teeth – and I have no teeth.'

Perhaps there is another side to the picture. I once much offended my own dentist (and it is a mistake to offend one's dentist while sitting in his chair) by remarking that dentists were the enemies of longevity. 'What do you mean by that?' he asked indignantly. 'Well,' I said, 'Nature plainly intended an old man to live on slops. You enable him to dig his grave with *your* teeth.'

Mr. Woodforde has written a fascinating book. His immense erudition is lightly worn.

Painlessly he takes us through the whole development of dentistry, shows its relevance to social life and manners, deals with modern techniques, relates it to forensic medicine, and indeed to every aspect of human existence. He has made a real contribution to history, or at least to those aspects of it which official historians so often forget.

JAMES LAVER

A Delicate Subject

Inhibitions to do with false teeth have a short history. The gold and bone appliances of ancient Etruria were luxuries to be admired; in eighteenth-century England sets of square ivory teeth were rich men's adornments: they resembled the real thing no more than periwigs real hair and, like periwigs, they were often removed. They came out at the dinner table.

Embarrassment dates from the nineteenth century. By about

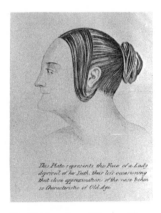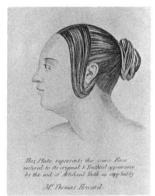

Frontispiece from Thomas Howard's On the Loss of Teeth, *1857.*

1840 laboured attempts at a natural appearance had brought false teeth into the category of the modern male toupee: however blatantly artificial, and loose, they had to be passed off as the work of Nature; however inconvenient for eating, they stayed in at meals.

The trials of wearers were made the more embarrassing by post-Regency puritanism which decreed it a vanity, like dyeing one's sidewhiskers, to resort to artificial teeth at all. Even the elderly Lord Palmerston did not escape criticism. In a political attack, Disraeli referred mockingly to Palmerston's false teeth and suggested that they 'would fall out of his mouth when speaking if he did not hesitate and halt so in his talk'.[1] How-

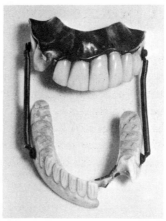

Typical early Victorian appliance – very unsafe for eating with, despite a degree of support that would be given by natural teeth still standing. The upper plate is gold with ivory teeth, the lower is carved ivory throughout.

ever, in ordinary polite society, propriety forbade any mention of false teeth. Wearers and beholders observed, as a dentist wrote regretfully, 'the most profound mystery'.[2]

Some wearers were sadly young: Willem, Prince of Orange, seems to have had a false set at nineteen, according to a letter by Queen Victoria dated 1859.[3] For the young lady with front teeth just pulled – probably by a local chemist – secrecy seemed so vital that she could not bring herself to ask where best to go for relief in her disfigurement. Instead she would read the

[1] Monypenny and Buckle, *Life of Disraeli*, 1929.
[2] W.H. Mortimer, *Essay on Artificial Teeth*, 1845.
[3] Roger Fulford, *Dearest Child*, 1964.

advertisements for Teeth More Natural Than Natural and become the prey of charlatans.

Although concealment of even a good practitioner's work was impossible, it remained for many a pathetic preoccupation. The Queen's dentist wrote of fitting a woman with a partial row of human teeth mounted on ivory, and of her return, four years later, with a sore mouth and the new teeth cemented to the natural ones with tartar: 'in her anxiety to keep her secret from every member of her family, she had never removed them'.[1] *The Dental Journal* for 1880 gives the case of a woman who called a doctor for a pain in the throat and did not divulge that she had swallowed her top set of teeth, a circumstance he luckily discovered for himself.

The extreme reticence enforced by propriety inhibited the Victorian novelists, despite their liking for lengthy descriptions of the person. Just as one might read all the works of Dickens or Thackeray without learning of the existence of prostitutes, so one might read a whole library of Victorian novels without learning that anyone's teeth were artificial. An occasional reference to fierceness was as much as convention would allow.

A certain delicacy seems to linger still in the minds of history and biography writers; they generally ignore the influence of teeth, whether false or natural, on social and public life and on the day-to-day habits of individuals. Yet this has been considerable. Oscar Wilde, to take one ninteenth-century figure, has been referred to as looking oddly furtive while telling his jokes. He looked furtive because he was ashamed of his teeth and put a hand in front of them:[2] a century earlier he might have screened his smiles with an ornamental fan.

Augustan wits of the eighteenth century avoided smiling altogether, and cultivated the dry ironic manner which flavours their writings; exposure of wretched mouths accorded ill with the urbanity and elegance of their speech. As for laughing, there was more than the sound it made behind the rule that true gentlemen should avoid it.

[1] Edwin Saunders, *Mineral Teeth*, 1841.
[2] William Rothenstein, painter. Quoted by Harold Nicolson, *Diaries and Letters*, 1967.

Victorian false teeth, more than anything else, lay behind the Victorian custom of eating in bedrooms just before dinner. It was a custom which insured against disaster at table as well as making possible the romantic affectation that young ladies lived on air. The hazards of mastication were real enough. Here is a passage from an 1846 textbook on dentistry:

> That it is a much easier task to make artificial teeth ornamental than useful, may be inferred from the fact that in by far the greater number of cases, they are much too insecure in the mouth to admit of any attempt at complete mastication of the food without displacement.[1]

Ornamental or not, in even lighthearted Victorian photographs people smile with closed lips.

Lack of dentistry as a factor in political history has been allowed due weight only by dentists. History books make nothing of the fact that Louis XIV and Queen Elizabeth I often had to give decisions while in agony; that Louis XIV, in particular, signed the Revocation of the Edict of Nantes while distraught with a tooth infection which had led to a sinus opening into the mouth and not healing;[2] that the wild judgements in later life of Gustavus Vasa, sixteenth-century King of Sweden, coincided with an appalling mouth condition: dentists who recently examined his skull, which was well preserved, found that decay in his lifetime had caused vast cavities, attrition and great loss of jawbone material.[3]

Only the specialist research papers of dentists consider the exhausting efforts of George Washington to improve his primitive false teeth and thereby his performance, or explain that President Grant's failure to address crowds during the world cruise of 1877 followed an accidental sweeping overboard of his false teeth.[4] Only in the limited dental world is it appreciated that without four teeth on a specially brief gold plate, made by a dentist later knighted, Sir Winston Churchill's war speeches might have been too slurred to rally

[1] Horatio Pass, *Artificial Teeth and Palates*, 1846.
[2] Arthur Lufkin, *A History of Dentistry.*   [3] Colin Davis, *Dental News*, 1967.
[4] Robert Hilkene, *Bulletin of the History of Dentistry*, Chicago, 1965.

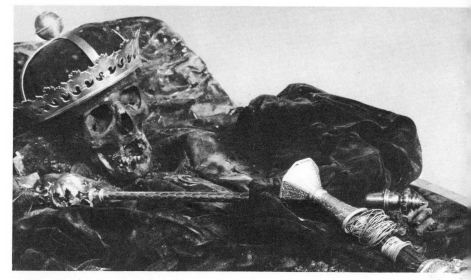

The skeleton of King Gustavus Vasa in Uppsala Cathedral, Sweden. He died in 1560 aged 64.

the spirits of the nation (the denture was made necessary by an accident in youth; Churchill kept all but five of his own teeth throughout a long life).

Mid-twentieth-century writers of memoirs have at least lightened the profound mystery with their amusing anecdotes – amusing, that is, in retrospect. Here is Sir Compton Mackenzie describing in *Octave Six* an abrupt crumbling of the façade of the late Sydney Dark, editor of the *Church Times*:

> He had dozed off in one of the armchairs of the Sandpit [at the Savile Club] with a lighted cigarette. Suddenly he leapt up with fumes coming from his mouth; that lighted cigarette had set fire to his false teeth. This is not just one more Savile story; I saw those fumes with my own eyes and I heard Sydney Dark's shout of dismay as he leapt up and hauled the denture out of his mouth.

Harold Macmillan writes in *Blasts of War* that a wartime mission to Finland began with comedy in that Lord Davies, his co-delegate, lost his false teeth on a Swedish train. He quotes a diary entry:

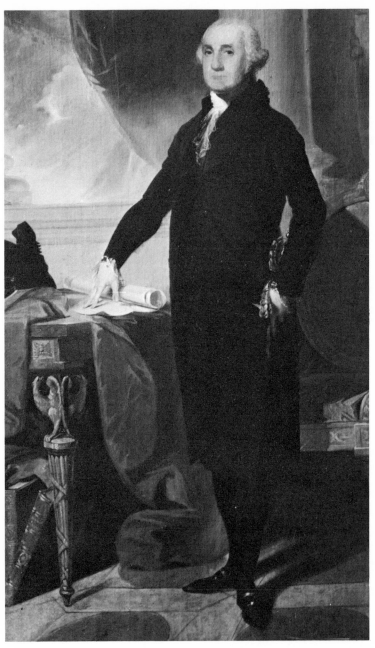

George Washington. Portrait by Gilbert Stuart, 1796.

As a director of the G.W.R. he is appealing to the Swedish Railway to give up his teeth, which he left in a sleeper. A search of an intense kind has been made . . . it is thought that the teeth may have been stolen by a Gestapo agent. [They were eventually recovered – unlike those of President Grant.]

But false teeth deserve more thoughtful treatment. The purpose of this book is to show them – and the lack of them – as a part of social history.

2

Dentistry of the Ancients

Poor teeth are often said to be caused by the effete foods of modern life, especially urban life. The theory has a long history. Two thousand years ago the Roman doctor Cornelius Celsus put it forward in his book *De Medicina*, advising 'the majority of inhabitants of cities and almost all literary men' to wash their mouths copiously on rising to prevent tooth decay: rude healthy people need not bother, as dental disease appeared to affect only those enjoying the idleness of civilization.

It is true that primitive peoples whose food needed energetic chewing had less trouble with their teeth; yet, even among these, decay was not uncommon many thousands of years ago. Evidence of it was once found, for instance, in seven skulls out of thirty-two dating from the Bronze Age.[1] One drawback to a diet of earth nuts, rye bread and raw meat and fish was the grit that came with it – particles of flint and shells – which sometimes wore away the grinding surfaces to the point where bacteria could enter the pulp of the teeth and cause abscesses.

The idea that civilized people tended to have much better teeth in the seventeenth and eighteenth centuries is disposed of by a visit to the National Portrait Gallery in London, where face after face is seen to be disfigured by missing teeth. A nuisance apparently brought on by the coarser food of those days was the formation of a cement-like tartar which gradually pushed back the gums until the teeth loosened. Thomas Berd-

[1] Maurice Smith, *A Short History of Dentistry*, 1958.

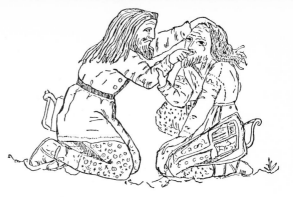

Drawing of a scene on a Phoenician vase found in Crimea.

more, dentist to George III, describes a bad case in his book *Disorders and Deformities of the Teeth* (1768):

> A gentleman of the Bank, not above twenty-three years of age, applied to me for advice concerning his Teeth . . . which gave him constant pain.
>
> I found them perfectly buried in Tartar, by which each set was united in one continuous piece, without any distinction, to show the interstices of the teeth, or their figure or size. The stony crust projected a great way over the gums on the inner side, as well as on the outer, and pressed upon them so hard as to have given rise to the pain he complained of. Its thickness at the upper surface was not less than half an inch. . . .

Toothache, theme of many a medieval gargoyle, has indeed troubled man throughout history. The Babylonians 5,000 years before Christ believed, like the Egyptians, that it was a manifestation of some divine displeasure; receipts circulated for its relief included prayers and incantations. The ancient Greeks used a mouthwash of castoreum and pepper and made pliers for pulling teeth out.

Aristotle (384–322 BC) urged caution over extractions, and said that having moved a tooth with the pliers, it was best to

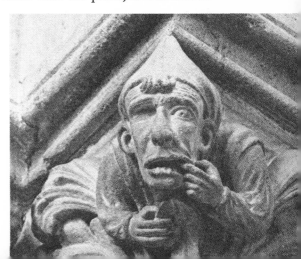

Man with toothache. Wells Cathedral.

extract it by hand, a method which must have greatly prolonged the patient's agony when the tooth was not already
loosened by gum disease. Celsus, 300 years later, offered
similar advice, and added that the first step was to detach the
gum all round.

Vanity rather than a wish to chew better almost certainly
inspired the first false teeth. The Greeks and the Phoenicians,

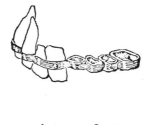

 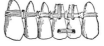

*Etruscan bridgework and Phoenician artificial teeth
wired to natural ones.*

who would bind loose teeth with gold wire, are known also to
have used ligatures for tying artificial ones to neighbouring
teeth. The Etruscans, however, excelled all at mechanical skill
with dental appliances. From finds made in Etruscan tombs, it
is certain that partial dentures of bridge-work type, serviceable
for mastication, were being worn in the district now called
Tuscany as early as 700 BC. Some were removable, others
permanently attached to natural teeth. Specimens are to be
seen in museums throughout Italy.

It was a usual Etruscan procedure to solder together wide
bands of pure gold which would fit over the natural teeth; the
substitute went into one of the bands and was held there by a
pin. Sometimes several teeth were fitted in this way. In the Civic
Museum of Tarquinia there is an appliance which carries three
false teeth; it is supported by five natural ones.

As the illustration shows, the gold bands were kept well above the gum line to prevent irritation, while the false teeth themselves rested not on the gums but on the flanking teeth. Dental craftsmanship of this order was not to reappear till the nineteenth century. The late Vincenzo Guerini, dental historian and an authority on dental remains in Italian museums, has suggested that Etruscans wore their false teeth proudly:

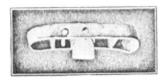

Etruscan appliance for supporting two inserted human teeth, one of which is missing. Civic Museum, Tarquinia.

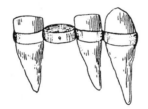

Etruscan appliance for supporting one inserted tooth, now missing. Conte Bruschi Museum, Tarquinia.

Since the gold bands of which they were constructed covered a considerable part of the crowns, they certainly could not have had the pretension of escaping notice, they being, on the contrary most visible. It is thus to be surmised that in those times the wearing of false teeth and other kinds of dental appliance was not a thing to be ashamed of; indeed that it rather constituted a luxury, a sort of refinement only accessible to persons of means.[1]

Non-mechanical dentistry in classical times was largely a mixture of folklore and popular belief; one remedy for tooth decay was a mouthwash made by boiling dogs' teeth in wine. Celsus said that toothache might be cured by applying to the

[1] Guerini, *A History of Dentistry*, 1909.

corresponding shoulder a plaster of myrrh, saffron, figs and mustard seed.

Pliny the Elder (AD 23–79), who wrote voluminously on natural history, recorded the contemporary belief that a frog tied to the jaws would make loose teeth firm; that pains in the gum responded to scratching with a tooth from a man who had met a violent death, and toothache to ear drops of the oil in which earthworms had been boiled. Equally absurd remedies, it may be said in passing, survived into the eighteenth century and beyond, when a frog tied to the neck was recommended by

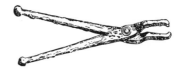

Roman pliers found in Saalburg Castle, Hamburg.

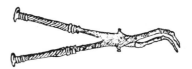

Roman pliers found at Pompeii.

physicians for a nose bleed and when sliced earthworms and snails formed the basis of a consumption remedy (as late as 1837 consumption and asthma would be treated with pills made of cobwebs).

The Romans did some ingenious work on partial sets of teeth, having probably learned much from the Etruscans who were now absorbed into the Roman Empire. Such dental replacements were by no means unusual. Horace (65–8 BC) describes in his eighth Satire two witches running so fast that the denture of one of them, Canidia, fell out. However, it must be assumed she had teeth of her own as well, for earlier in the same Satire Horace writes of her and the other witch, Sagana (who wore a wig), having torn a lamb to pieces with their teeth.

Martial (AD 40–104) alludes in several of his Epigrams to artificial teeth of bone and ivory. He praises Laecania, a courtesan, for having teeth as white as snow, but hastens to remark that they are not natural: 'Thais' teeth are black, Laecania's snowy white. How is that? One has her own, the other those you buy.'

He also refers to wooden teeth: 'Maxima has three teeth, all of which are boxwood and as black as pitch.' That some kind of easily removable denture could be had is suggested by a line addressed to a lady called Galla: 'And you lay aside your teeth at night as you do your silken dress.'

Whether the Romans made full as well as partial sets of false teeth remains uncertain. Guerini thought it probable. Their ability to carry out crown work is proved by the find at Satricum of a gold cap made to fit over a defective lower front tooth.

Unfortunately Celsus and others who wrote about the treatment of dental diseases did not allude to the mechanical substitutes in use. They were not concerned with such things any more than medical writers of today are normally concerned to write about wigs and monocles.

Certainly the Romans attached importance to dental integrity. An article in the Law of the Twelve Tables sets out penalties for violence causing damage to the teeth: 'Whoever shall cause the tooth of a free man to be knocked out shall pay a fine of three hundred *as*, that of a slave one hundred and fifty.'

3

The First European False Teeth

If full upper and lower sets of false teeth were ever made by the Romans, they probably resembled the perfunctory hinged appliance illustrated. It was dug up in Switzerland and dates from the late fifteenth century, according to the German medical historian Gernot Rath.[1] By then, he says, half-hearted

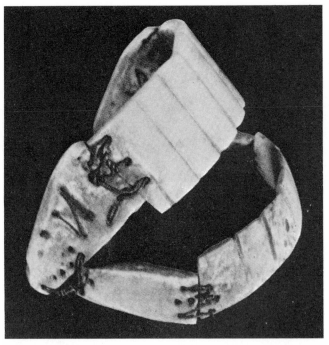

Full upper and lower set dating from about 1500 dug up in Switzerland.

[1] *Aus der Geschichte des Zahnersatzes*, 1958.

14

mouth decorations of this sort were occasionally acquired by Continental women; they would pull them out at the beginning of a meal and with great dexterity slip them back whenever there was a pause in the eating.

For hundreds of years after the collapse of the Roman Empire – so it can be sweepingly stated – all kinds of dental skill deteriorated in Europe. The writings of a Persian physician called Rhazes (850–923) make the next landmark. Rhazes was one of the first people to recommend filling cavities; though his stoppings of alum and mastic cannot have been hard enough to last long.

Abulcasis (1050–1122), an Arabian surgeon, illustrates and describes dental scrapers for the first time in *De Chirurgia*, a work which remained for centuries a standard surgical text-book. It shows fourteen scrapers and sets the scene for their use:

> Sometimes on the surface of the teeth, both inside and outside, are deposited rough ugly-looking scales, black, green and yellow; this corruption is communicated to the gums, and the teeth are in process of time denuded. Lay the patient's head on your lap and scrape the teeth and molars. . . .

Abulcasis still counsels the slow extraction method of Celsus, starting with loosening the gums. One must avoid, he says, acting like the ignorant tooth-drawing barbers who often cause great injury. Get your patient's head firmly between your knees, grip the bad tooth between finger and thumb, or with the pliers, and shake it methodically from side to side. The ignorant barbers, with a speedier method, at least made extraction without pain killers a less dreadful experience.

Abulcasis gives detailed instructions about binding loose teeth to firm ones with gold wire. He deals with false teeth in a line or two, simply observing that gaps left by lost teeth may be filled with bone substitutes bound in the same way.

The great French surgeon Guy de Chauliac (1309–68), has a long section on dentistry in his *Chirurgia Magna*, but offers hardly anything that was not said by Abulcasis 250 years earlier. He covers the subject of artificial teeth as dismissively as Abulcasis and in almost the same terms.

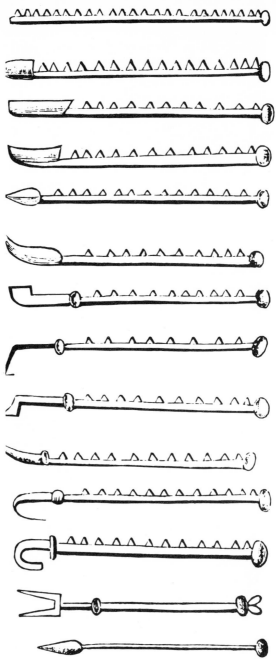

Set of fourteen dental scrapers illustrated by Abulcasis.

16

Some progress is indicated a century later by the records of Arculanus (1412–84), an Italian university professor. He makes the first known reference to gold leaf as a filling material – one that had to be pressed in laboriously little by little. This procedure was still sometimes used in the early twentieth century.

In fifteenth-century England barber-surgeons – the main drawers of teeth – were becoming common: they had been

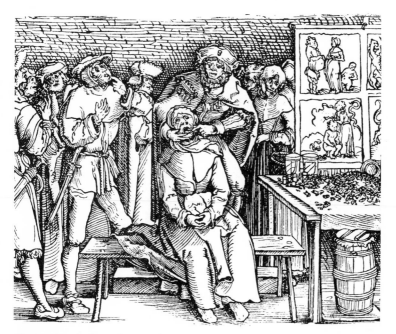

Market-place dentistry. Seventeenth century.

formed in 1308 into a guild which was not finally disbanded till 1745. There were also plenty of itinerant tooth-drawers, mostly ignorant impostors, who liked to wear necklaces of teeth or to sew them on their belts. They were a popular attraction at markets and fairs, their presence signalled by loud music which also served to drown the cries of the patients. The sales talk of these people about painless extraction gave rise to the once popular adage 'to lie like a tooth-drawer'.

The principal tooth-pulling instruments were pliers (forceps), pelicans and elevators. The pelican, so named from the fancied resemblance of its claw to the bird's beak, came into use when little progress was being made with the pliers. The claw prised the tooth out sideways, purchase coming from the serrated fulcrum which was squarely applied to the outer gum.

The elevator could be useful for the final removal. After pushing its tapering blade between the root of the bad tooth

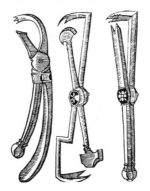

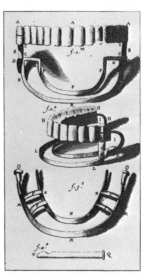

Two pelicans and a pair of curved pincers. Sixteenth century.

Fauchard upper sets for mouths where all lower teeth are still present.

and the one next to it, the operator would make a turning movement calculated to lift the root clear.

In view of the alarming observations of contemporary surgeons about the danger of extraction, it is not surprising that thinking people greatly feared the operation, and that only the worst toothache would make them undergo it. Ambrose Paré (1517–92), surgeon to the French Court, and now known as the father of modern surgery, wrote that in pulling out a tooth too violently there was a risk of dislocating the jaw, bringing part of it away, and concussion of the brain and eyes. And any such mishap might be followed by fever, apostema, abundant haemorrhage or death.

Great skill, he says, is needed for using the pelican, for otherwise it will almost certainly happen that several good teeth will be knocked out instead of the one intended. He tells the story of a tooth-drawer's young servant who found an opportunity, when his master was at table, to try his hand with a pelican, and managed to relieve a villager of three perfectly sound teeth. To quieten the man's loud complaints, he told him his master might come out and make him pay for three teeth instead of one. The master did come out, and the poor man hurried away – with three teeth in his pouch and the one that hurt him still in his mouth.

Queen Elizabeth I suffered badly from tooth decay and knew only too well the misery of extraction. A passage in John Strype's *Life of Bishop Aylmer* (1701), describes an occasion when it became necessary:

> It was in the Month of December 1578, when she was so excessively tormented with that Distemper [toothache] that she had no Intermission Day or Night, and it forced her to pass whole Nights without taking any Rest; and came to that Extremity, that her Physicians were called in and consulted. . . . The pulling it out was esteemed by all the safest way; to which, however, the Queen, as was said, was very averse, as afraid of the acute Pain that accompanied it. And now it seems it was that the Bishop of London being present, a Man of high Courage, persuaded her that the pain was not so much, and not at all to be dreaded; and to convince her thereof told her, she should have a sensible Experience of it in himself, though he were an old man, and had not many Teeth to spare; and immediately had the Surgeon come and pull out one of his Teeth, perhaps a decayed one, in her Majestie's Presence. Which accordingly was don: and She was hereby encouraged to submit to the Operation herself.

In England at this time the wearing of artificial teeth was extremely rare. When the Queen eventually lost her front teeth, she made occasional use, for appearance sake, of a device that can have been effective only when she did not open her mouth. Herbert Norris in *Costume and Fashion* quotes a contemporary's description in 1602:

> The Queen is still . . . frolicy and merry, only her face showeth some decay, which to conceal when she cometh in public she putteth many fine cloths into her mouth to bear out her cheeks. . . .

Similar lip padding was used 200 years later by George Washington while having a portrait painted.

At the French Court, restorative dentistry was more sophisticated. Henry III (once a suitor of Elizabeth) had recourse to several front teeth made of bone. According to Norris, he was unusually vain, colouring his face and eyes and even his ears. Prematurely bald as a result of trying to dye his hair, he wore either a wig or a turban. Arthur Lufkin in *A History of Dentistry* quotes a traveller's account of watching the morning ritual of fitting Henry's false teeth:

> I thought that the rubbing of the lips would be the last ceremony, but instantly I saw another servant kneel before the patient, take hold of his beard and pull down the lower jaw; then, having moistened the finger in I do not know what kind of water, in a little glass vessel, he took a certain white powder with which he rubbed the gums and teeth; then opening a little bottle he took out some small things of bone – I do not know what – and fastened them with fine wire to the adjoining teeth on either side.

Tongue play with teeth thus lightly adjusted must have been irresistible: Norris writes that it was reported of Henry that his mouth was always twitching.

In Britain till at least the end of the seventeenth century progress in dentistry was negligible – less than that in France and elsewhere on the Continent. The need for treatment was undoubtedly great. The diet of the well-to-do included a preponderance of sugary cakes and marzipan sweetmeats; and even meat pies would be topped with a mixture that included a mass of sugar and rosewater. Shakespeare, whose writings show him to have been sensitive to bad smells, made numerous references to 'stinking breath'. There were recipes for mouthwashes to help mask this inevitable companion to dental decay. Thomas Vicary's *The English Man's Treasure*, 1613, offered the following advice:

> To take away the stinking of the mouth – wash mouthe with water and vinegar and chew masticke then wash mouthe with the decoction of Annis seeds, mints and cloves sodden in wine.

Vicary's credentials are impressive. He appears on the title

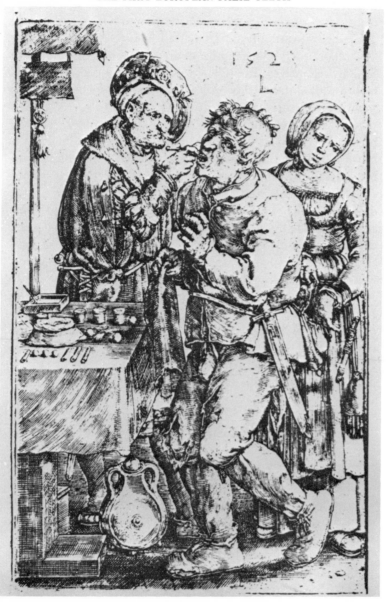

At a market. The elegantly dressed dentist has decorated the upturned brim of his hat with teeth. One notes a woman trying to steal the patient's money. An engraving made in 1523 by Lucas van Leydon of Holland, 1494–1533.

page of his book as: 'Sergeant Chirurgion to King Henry the 8. To King Edward the 6. To Queen Marie. And to our late Soveraigne Lady Queene Elizabeth. Also Chiefe Chirurgion to St. Bartholomewes Hospitall.' No doubt many people tried his mouthwash of stamped pepper and warm red wine for expelling the worms then thought to cause toothache.

Apart from extraction, the chief dental operation of even the best barber-surgeons was cleaning. There were no tooth-brushes for home use; though some people used toothpicks or bits of cloth. The barber-surgeon scraped the teeth with various metal instruments and then rubbed them over with a stick dipped in *aqua fortis* – that is, a solution of nitric acid. This certainly made the sound ones white, but only for as long as the enamel held out. The damage done by repeated use of acid cleaners – still resorted to as recently as the eighteenth century – was of course irreparable and in due course fatal to the teeth. A whitener recommended by Sir Hugh Platt in *Delightes for Ladies* was at least safe: a quart of honey, a quart of vinegar and a pint of wine boiled together, to be used at intervals as the teeth become stained.

A little book called *The Jewel House of Art and Nature* (1653), contains a warning about having teeth cleaned at the barber's:

> And here by those miserable examples that I have seen in some of my nearest friends, I am inforced to admonish all men to be careful, how they suffer their teeth to be made white with aqua fortis, which is the Barber's usual water; for unless the same be well delayed, and carefully applied, a man with a few dressings, may be driven to borrow a rank of teeth.

The author recommended a dentifrice (contemporary word) formed by mingling finely powdered alabaster with a jelly, the substance to be made up into little rolls four to five inches long. The notion of anyone being *obliged* to acquire a rank of teeth would have amused his readers.

In a 1654 treatise on surgery, Peter Lowe wrote of artificial teeth being made of ivory and whale-bone and fastened with a wire, but admitted, 'I am not mindful to insist on this practice as I might, because it is seldom practised'.

The first English book solely on dentistry, *The Operator for the Teeth* (1685), by Charles Allen of York, is hardly more encouraging about false teeth:

> When our decay'd Teeth are so far gone before we think of any Remedy for their preservation, that whatever we do proves fruitless: and that notwithstanding all our best endeavours they . . . quite rot away, or that some intolerable pain has made us draw them: we are not yet to despair, and esteem ourselves Toothless for the rest of our Life; the loss indeed is great, but not irreparable, there is still some help for it; the natural want may be supplied artificially.

Artificial substitutes, he goes on to suggest, may possibly help to keep the teeth next to them firmer and stronger.

Allen deplores a practice known as transplantation, extracting rotten teeth or stumps and putting into their sockets sound ones drawn from another person's head – 'it is only robbing Peter to pay Paul'; but he considers it 'very profitable and advantageous' to transplant the teeth of brutes like sheep and dogs into the human jaw. However, from the vagueness of his instructions for doing this, it need not be supposed that either Allen or anyone else ever carried it out.

As in Roman days, the poets made occasional cheerful references to false teeth. *Love's Labour's Lost* has the line: 'This is the flower that smiles on everyone, to show his teeth as white as whale's bone.' Robert Herrick (1591–1674), author of the poem 'Gather Ye Rosebuds', was apparently amused to see a man with several front teeth made, in his opinion, from part of a bone handle. In the epigram *Upon Glasco* he writes:

> Glasco had none, but now some teeth has got;
> Which though they furre, will neither ake, or rot.
> Six teeth he has, whereof twice two are known
> Made of a Haft, that was a mutton-bone.
> Which not for use, but meerly for the sight,
> He wears all day, and draws those teeth at night.

4

Measuring the Mouth with Compasses

In 1664 Samuel Pepys's wife had her teeth 'new done' by one Peter de la Roche, who made them 'pretty handsome': de la Roche is believed to have been the first of London's Operators for the Teeth, men who made themselves specialists in dental work. Some had scraped and pulled teeth as pupils of barber-surgeons; others had experience as goldsmiths and ivory turners.

By the end of the seventeenth century they were beginning to realize that the highest rewards could come from supplying the rich with false teeth. Advertisements began to appear in the public press; an early one from *The Ladies' Diary* of 1711 runs as follows:[1]

> Artificial teeth set in so well as to eat with them, and not to be distinguish'd from natural, not to be taken out at night, as is by some falsely suggested, but may be worn for years together. They are an ornament to the mouth and greatly help the speech. Also, teeth clean'd and drawn, by John Watts (Operator) who applies himself wholly to the said business, and lives in Racquet Court, in Fleet Street, London.

Ivory from the hippopotamus or walrus was the normal material for making artificial teeth and the bases to carry them. If the job was just a row of front teeth, a single piece of ivory carved in representation would be fastened to the existing teeth on either side with a thread of metal or silk. Since the ligature was difficult for the wearer to tie and untie by himself, the piece

[1] J. Menzies Campbell, *Dentistry Then and Now*, 1963.

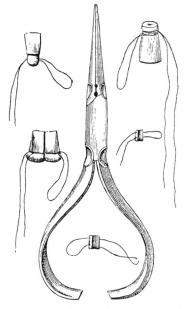

Pincers used by Fauchard for tying in artificial teeth, human or ivory, with gold wire.

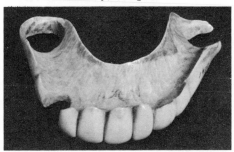

Upper piece which probably had enough support from three natural teeth to be tolerably secure. Eighteenth century.

would seldom leave the mouth, and thereby cause all kinds of discomfort.

Teeth not fixed with threads, which *could* be taken out at night, and properly cleaned, are referred to in 1718 in a book by the German surgeon, Lorenz Heister (1683–1758). He writes of partial sets made of either the ivory or the tusks of a hippopotamus which were kept in position in the gap between standing teeth simply by their form. He does not go into detail, taking the line that making false teeth is outside the sphere of the general surgeon.

That false teeth of any kind were not yet regarded very seriously – in England, anyway – is clear from the toothlessness apparent in eighteenth-century portraits. But though application to John Watts might have filled sitters' lips out, the typical rows of teeth procurable in those days did not necessarily do much to correct a facial disfigurement: sometimes they made it worse by enforcing an unnatural position of the lower jaw. (A portrait painter working on the poet William Wordsworth thought dentures were causing distortion, and asked him to take them out for some of the preliminary sketches.)

John Watts, whose advertisement has been quoted, was the founder of a famous firm of Operators for the Teeth which specialized in false teeth and continued in business for about 150 years. William Green, who joined the firm in 1744, was appointed Operator for the Teeth to George II; the whiteness of false teeth made by him is celebrated in a verse by Charles Churchill, quoted in Chapter 18.

Thomas Berdmore joined in 1760 and was appointed to look after the teeth of George III. He was an exceptional operator. His book on the teeth and gums (1768), with a long section on false teeth, remained for years the only English textbook on dentistry. It was widely translated and stayed in print till 1844. John Hunter's *The Natural History of the Human Teeth* (1771) was not a serious rival. Hunter was a brilliant surgeon and anatomist: the only branch of practical dentistry on which he could write from personal experience was transplantation – a subject dealt with in a separate chapter.

Berdmore writes as follows about the kind of false teeth then most usual, the partial set tied in semi-permanently with thread:

> Although artificial Teeth are evidently ornamental; although they give a healthy juvenile air to the countenance, improve the tone

of the voice, render pronunciation more agreable and distinct, help mastication, and preserve the opposite Teeth from growing prominent; yet many are prejudiced against them on account of some inconveniences . . . they are said . . . Not to sit easy on the gums: – Seldome to stand firm: – And to loosen after some time the neighbouring Teeth to which they are fastened. – Or, the hard ligature, which is commonly used, is often seen to cut very deep into sound Teeth. . . .

Berdmore drew much of his income from false teeth, but is honest enough to admit that neighbouring teeth are damaged and loosened. Advising silk and not wire, he continues:

Can the consideration of such a loss justly outweigh the obvious advantages of artificial Teeth? Or, is it a matter of great concern, if a man once in five or six years is obliged to have one added to the number of his artificial Teeth?

Full lower dentures were laboriously carved in one piece and looked roughly like modern ones; they would be weighted to help gravity keep them on the gums. Full upper sets were not seriously attempted. There had to be for anchorage at least two existing teeth near the front or, failing that, one tooth augmented by a stump of one that would take in its root a post attached to the denture.

Lacking a reliable wax for the job, operators could not take a full impression. They got to work after observing the mouth and measuring it with compasses. Fitting was done by painting the gums with a colour, then repeatedly letting down the set of teeth in trial and scraping the parts of the ivory base which picked up colour. If the patient was lucky, something of a fit would be achieved – for the time being.

The poorness of the fits tolerated is indicated by the existence of practitioners supplying false teeth to unseen patients. One of the first was a French silversmith called Pilleau, practising in London, whose advertisements in the 1730s may have appealed to shy provincials. He sent directions for moulding a piece of wax into a horseshoe shape, and then pressing it on to the jaws in such a way that standing teeth pierced it and made an impression of the gums on either side. From this crude record in soft wax he set to work. A British-born London operator, Gamaliel Voice, advertised as follows:

> Those that are at a distance, and have not opportunity of coming to town, may be furnished with any number [of teeth] that are quite out in front if the rest be fast; and this may be done by sending a pattern, which he will direct them to do if they please send a letter to him, paying the carriage by post or otherwise.

False teeth ordered by post must often have been excruciating to wear. Letters preserved show they were sometimes returned at once to the maker with agitated instructions for alteration.

In the better or, at any rate, the more expensive sets, human teeth were incorporated by cutting them off at the neck and pinning them into prepared sockets on the front of the denture base. They came from graveyards and battlefields and from poor people willing to sacrifice teeth for money. This list of charges payable in 1781 to Paul Jullion of 47 Gerrard Street, London, shows the price difference between human and artificial replacements:[1]

> Constructing and fitting an artificial tooth with silken ligatures 10s. 6d.
> Fitting a human tooth (on the same construction as an artificial one) with silken ligatures £2 2s.
> Constructing and fitting an upper or an under row of artificial teeth without fastenings £10 10s.
> Fitting an upper or under row or human teeth, without fastenings £31 10s.

Where expense was no object, teeth of silver, mother of pearl or enamelled copper could be ordered for attaching to an ivory base. The Duchess of Portland, in a letter of 1735, describes the exquisitely dressed and foppish Lord Hervey, hitherto toothless, appearing one day with 'the finest set of Egyptian pebble teeth that ever you saw'. John, Lord Hervey, vice-chamberlain to Queen Caroline, was at this time thirty-nine. His false teeth are believed to have been of agate and made in Italy.[2]

But even the finest sets of teeth had an awkwardness at their

---

[1] Menzies Campbell.   [2] *The Life and Correspondence of Mrs. Delaney*, 1861.

necks which meant they were presentable only when partially veiled by the lips; the eye was otherwise arrested either by a gap below the natural gums or by the yellow strip of ivory into which the substitutes were riveted. With uncertain adaptation to the jaws, and primitive fastening arrangements, false teeth were in general almost useless for eating. Except for the unself-conscious, who liked them as ornaments, they long remained a comment-causing luxury that was better left alone. As late as 1789 a *Morning Post* advertisement could imply they were something of a new invention:[1]

> TEETH. How mortifying and disagreable it must be to those that are unfortunate in their loss; and how agreable and pleasing it must be to them in finding, that they may have the defect supplied with others, from a single tooth to a whole set, on very moderate terms . . . made to fix in quite firm, without any pain or danger of their ever coming out through accident. . . .

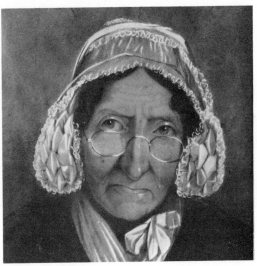

Eighteenth–nineteenth-century woman in need of false teeth. Marie Tussaud, founder of Madame Tussaud's Museum in London, 1760–1850.

In reality the bad appearance of missing or defective teeth was so much an accepted evil that dentists had to work hard

[1] Menzies Campbell.

to sell treatment that went beyond first aid. No one wrote more convincingly on the subject than Berdmore; he urged the careless to remember that no one could excel in the art of pleasant conversation 'whose loss of teeth, or rotten livid stumps, and fallen lips and hollow cheeks destroy . . . the happy expression of the countenance'.

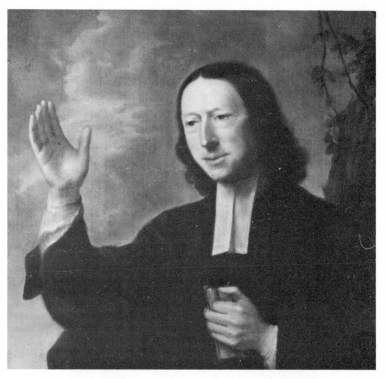

Eighteenth-century man in need of false teeth, John Wesley, 1703–91.

A practitioner called Martin van Butchell was not content with the printed word for stimulating sales of his false teeth ('useful ornaments', he called them, 'most helpful to enunciation'); he went all out for personal publicity. In the 1770s he could be seen riding about London on a white pony painted sometimes with purple spots and sometimes with black ones. Numerous visitors were attracted to his house in Mount Street

by his keeping there, in the sitting room, the embalmed body
of his first wife.

Lord Chesterfield, advising constant washing of the teeth in
the widely read *Letters to His Son* (published 1774, a year after
his death), undoubtedly had an effect:

> A dirty mouth has real ill consequences to the owner, for it
> infallibly causes the decay, as well as the intolerable pain of the
> teeth; and it is very offensive to his acquaintance, for it will most
> inevitably stink.

(His own teeth, he told his son, were falling out for want of care
when he was young.)

Lord Hervey, setting a good example with his hygienic
pebble teeth, reports in *Memoirs of the Reign of George II* that the
king said Bishop Hoadly had 'nasty rotten teeth'; and the wife
of Sir Horace Walpole[1] was as 'offensive to the nose and ears',
according to Hervey, 'as to the eye'. Lord Chief Justice Ryder,
enduring a hollow tooth in his twenties, was 'very uneasy in
company', fearing he had 'a stinking breath and it was perceived'.[2]

Elizabeth Burton puts it forward in *The Georgians at Home*
that the fan was a very necessary piece of equipment in those
days. Apart from its normal fanning and flirtatious function, it
could be used to hide a smile which displayed squalid teeth, or
as a screen to protect the nose against mephitic breath. Without
a liberal sprinkling, or sucking, of civet, musk, ambergris and
other strong essences, no room full of people was likely to
remain habitable for long.

However, Horace Walpole, letter-writer nephew of Sir
Horace, is able to say at fifty-two that periodical dissolving of
alum in the mouth 'has so fortified my teeth that they are as
strong as the pen of Junius'. He was commiserating with
George Montagu over 'the vacancy that has occurred in your
mouth'.

---

[1] Brother of Sir Robert Walpole.
[2] His *Diary*, quoted by Elizabeth Burton, *The Georgians at Home*, 1967.

5

The Tooth-drawers

In Hogarth's Electioneering pictures, which clearly show eighteenth-century people with their mouths open, almost everyone over the age of twenty-five seems badly lacking in teeth. For all but a handful of the population, extraction was the only form of dentistry ever encountered. Masticators, resembling large nut-crackers and designed to pre-crush an intended mouthful of food, had a limited sale among the toothless – and were still to be had at the end of the nineteenth century.

Attempts at stopping teeth was exotic treatment for which molten lead or gutta percha was used. In the latter part of the eighteenth century, fillings were occasionally undertaken with gold foil pressed in tediously and painfully bit by bit, an ancient procedure capable of making a good repair if there was no leakage and a minimum of decay remaining below. From the 1830s an unstable and dangerous amalgam of mercury and silver scrapings, slapped home in a minute, found plenty of takers who were soon sorry. A balanced amalgam of the kind used today did not appear till 1895. Modern gold inlays date from 1890.

Till at least 1800 any barber invariably combined hair-cutting with both tooth-extraction and blood-letting. According to the poet John Gay (1685–1732):

> His pole with pewter basons hung
> Black rotten teeth in order strung,
> Rang'd cups, that in the window stood,

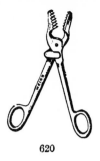

620

620 John Weiss & Son's Masticator (White's Patent).

Invaluable to all persons with defective teeth.
This instrument works on the principle of the action of the teeth. Meat and other food which requires masticating is easily and quickly prepared for digestion by the aid of the Masticator.

The food when ready for eating is first cut up into small pieces, which are then crushed with the Masticator into a pulp easily swallowed. The instrument is best worked if held almost horizontally with BOTH hands. To avoid chilling the food, dip the blades from time to time into hot water.

After use care must be taken to thoroughly cleanse the Masticator in hot water with a brush, and to rub it dry with a piece of chamois leather. It can be easily taken apart for the purpose of cleansing.

Best Electro-plated £0 12 6

Neat Cases are charged extra.

A dental supplier's catalogue entry c. 1880. Masticators were occasionally recommended at the end of recipes in cookery books.

> Lin'd with red rags to look like blood,
> Did well his threefold trade explain,
> Who shav'd, drew teeth, and breath'd a vein.

In country districts tooth-drawing was carried out by such tradesmen as blacksmiths and shoemakers, who found it a useful

33

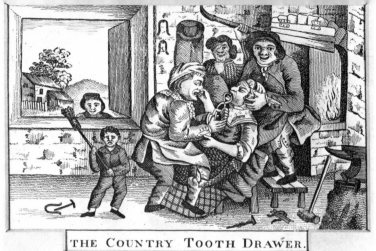

THE COUNTRY TOOTH DRAWER.

A tooth-drawing farrier uses both hands to grip his pincers. The countrywoman patient grabs his nose. Caricature after Dighton. c. 1785.

sideline. Parson Woodforde, the diarist, in 1776 recorded having to call in the village farrier to extract a tooth for him. There was also the itinerant operator of the market place and fair, announcing his presence and drowning cries by having an assistant to beat a drum or blow a trumpet. Only fifty years ago he would still be met with occasionally in remote districts. The market-place operator may be seen to this day in Morocco, performing with dash before an appreciative audience.

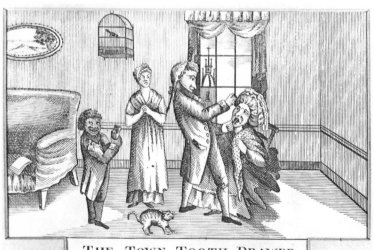

THE TOWN TOOTH DRAWER.

A bag-wigged dentist operating with a tooth key. A black boy in livery stands by with case of instruments. Caricature after Dighton. c. 1785.

Apothecaries and chemists drew teeth; and country doctors often felt obliged to do so. The Rev. Francis Kilvert, in his *Diary*, records chatting over a hedge on a May evening in 1875 with one William Hulbert who had just

been to the doctor and had seven teeth and stumps ('snags', he called them) pulled out, and whilst the doctor was pulling out the

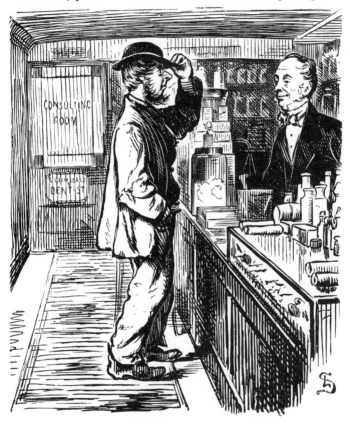

A STOPPER.

Itinerant Vendor. "GIE US A CHRIS'MAS-BOX, GUVNOR! I ALLUS HAS MY TEETH DRAWED 'ERE."

Practitioner. "ALL RIGHT, MY MAN! STEP INSIDE, AND I'LL TAKE ONE OUT FOR NOTHING."   *[Itinerant Vendor does not seem to see the pull of it.*

The apothecary-dentist. Punch, *1870.*

teeth he felt three tumours (he called them 'knubs') in Hulbert's head. These he insisted on cutting out on the spot. and Hulbert brought the whole lot, 'snags' and 'knubs', home in his pocket. 'It made I sweat', he said. 'It was all over in ten minutes, but the place was like a butcher's shop and once I should have liked to knock the doctor through the door.'

Fashionable doctors preferring, among other things, not to expose themselves to the possibility of personal attack, avoided dental work. An article in *The Forceps* (published fortnightly between 1844 and 1845) stated:[1]

> A pure surgeon . . . can scarcely be expected to pay any attention to a subject of such minor importance as the teeth, or soil his aristocratic fingers by touching a key instrument. . . .

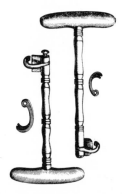

Two key instruments with changeable hooks. Eighteenth century.

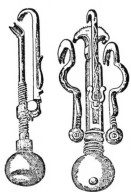

Two pelicans. Eighteenth century.

By the 1770s the key had become the most popular extraction tool. Its mechanical leverage, like that of the pelican, was designed to make the job rapid – a matter of importance at a time when no local anaesthetic existed. With claw engaged over the crown, a brisk turn was theoretically enough to dislocate the tooth from its socket; but the consequences could be vicious. On the Continent as well as in England the key was used till well into the nineteenth century, largely superseding the forceps.

[1] Menzies Campbell.

36

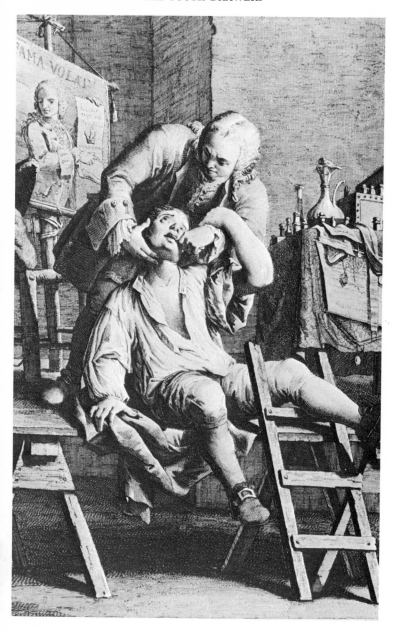

Market-place extraction. Maggiotto. Eighteenth century.

The most usual posture for having teeth drawn was sitting or lying on the floor; operators liked the convenience of being able to grip the head between their knees. However, towards the end of the eighteenth century the more sophisticated ones put patients in some kind of chair (operating chairs were rare till the mid nineteenth century). The French dentist, Pierre Fauchard, who sometimes proffered a comfortable sofa, had exerted some influence by protesting in a book[1] that the

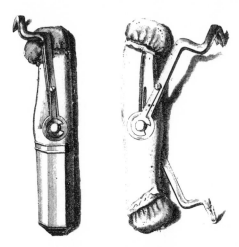

Fauchard's single and double pelican. Eighteenth century. Note the changeable hooks.

floor position, besides being uncomfortable, was indecent and unnecessarily alarming, especially to the pregnant.

But whatever the patient's position, it often happened that both parties would be involved in a scene of indignity. Charles Bew, a dentist who served the Prince Regent at Brighton, describes several such scenes with evident enjoyment.[2] One eminent practitioner, he writes, was 'overbalanced by a fear-excited effort of his patient' (who was on the ground) and 'precipitated from his posterior station to one more prominent on the carpet than suited the gravity of his calling or disposition'.

An 'apothecary-dentist of Shropshire', who stood on a chair

[1] *Le Chirurgien Dentiste*, 1728.   [2] *Diseases in the Teeth and Gums*, 1819.

to operate on a seated client, was 'thrown to the ground by a convulsive plunge' and 'narrowly escaped a fractured skull'. Bew himself often had difficulties. His zestful style in describing them may be attributable to his having been an actor until he took up dentistry:

> A pilot's wife (at Dover), whose rotundity of habit would have caused twenty stone to kick the beam, was pained and alarmed to agitation with the toothache. Anguish and argument together succeeding, a *trial* for *ejectment* proved fortunately successful: but as the annoying tooth was in the act of resigning possession, under the pressure of the instrument, my portly patient, whose ruddy arm encircled my neck, either actuated by alarm or extacy, so far lost her self-possession, as to throw herself upon me; whereby my half-genuflected position proving insufficient for the *weight* of such an honour, the affair was happily finished by the *flooring* of patient and practitioner; and, though least in the joyous scene of success, I had nearly suffered suffocation from rapture.

The consequences are 'ever more or less disastrous', says Bew, 'when the hands of the patient are *snatchingly* applied to those of the operator at the critical moment. . . .' At a boarding school where he attended

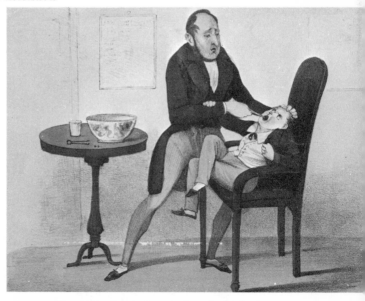

Incompetent first aid by the schoolmaster. One of an early nineteenth-century series of prints called Arithmetical Sketches.

the children were imprudently placed in a corner of the apartment, like so many encircled lambs for the impending slaughter. Previous to my appearance, a chair had been placed in the middle of the room, and by its side a table loaded with basons, jugs of water, tumblers, towels, and the paraphernalia of operation.

The first who took her station was a parlour boarder. . . . All went well till the critical moment of removal; when seizing the instrument with both hands, and, as if they were insufficient to *stay proceedings*, the feet flew up to their aid; and, coming in contact with the leaf of the table, overturned it and the contents . . . the discordant shrieks which succeeded the *crash*, from all the party spontaneously joining chorus, resembled the yell of an Indian horde, dispersed by the explosion of a bombshell or a Congreve rocket.

Bew writes as follows of an extra-nervous woman patient:

The honourable sister of a worthy deceased baron sent for me . . . for the extraction of a tooth; and, after detaining me *three hours* with details of the causes which made her a coward, pertinaciously resisted all attempts at removal; till, wrought by pain and the reproaches of her family, an hysterical affection suppressed further resistance, and the tooth was extracted under temporary aberration of intellect.

Another patient, a major-general this time, who was equipped 'with every manly and virtuous feeling . . . absolutely bound me by word of honour not to take out the tooth till he gave me permission; although the instrument was on the tooth, and taken off half a dozen times previous to its extraction'.

In the eighteenth-century *Memoirs of William Hickey* there is a gruesome story of a young man who tried with misplaced

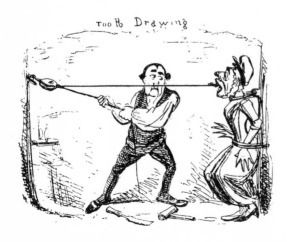

Tooth Drawing

Home tooth-drawing. Early nineteenth century.

courage to be his own tooth-drawer. Unable to get a surgeon
to visit him at once, and maddened with pain, he

> swore he would extract it [the aching tooth] himself or drive it
> down his throat. He took up a large carving knife and with the
> point thereof dreadfully lacerated and hacked his gums, after
> which he attempted with the handle of the knife to beat out the
> offending tooth, in doing which he materially injured the lower
> jaw, producing a severe and dangerous inflammation; so bad did
> it become that during upwards of four months he had three
> surgeons in close attendance upon him, they being several times
> apprehensive of mortification and of a locked jaw, large splinters
> of bone daily working through the wound. . . . He however
> ultimately recovered, with leaving only an immense scar on the
> outside of his neck. . . .

George III was a self-possessed patient according to an
account (admiringly written up by Bew) of the preliminaries to
a successful tooth-drawing:

> A tooth which had for some time annoyed his Majesty, was
> condemned to extraction: the dentist of the household was com-
> manded to attend. On his introduction by the page in waiting, the
> Sovereign, with his accustomed good-humoured condescension
> (feeling the probability of the first professional visit producing
> alarm in the operator), said, 'I don't know whether *you* are afraid
> of *me*; but I can tell you, *I am* afraid of *you*.' The dentist bowing
> replied, he hoped all would go well. – 'Oh, I dare say,' said the
> Sovereign; 'but I think it would go better with me, if I have a
> little *brandy*.' – 'After the operation, I presume.' – 'No, before,'
> replied his Majesty, 'to give me courage.' – The spirit being
> brought, the page was about to present it. 'No, no,' exlaimed the
> King, 'let the dentist do it – he makes me a coward; let him give
> me courage.' The brandy was accordingly poured out, and
> presented by the dentist; to whom his Majesty, smiling as he
> refused it, replied, 'I have no need of it; but was merely anxious
> to observe if your hand was steady.'

6

Powders and Tinctures

Before anaesthetics, it was not uncommon for tooth-drawers to immobilize seated patients with leather straps. The hope of avoiding such an encounter promoted a ready sale for the powders and tinctures advertised in every newspaper for the relief, or prevention, of the universal scourge of toothache; sufferers would try almost anything before submitting themselves to the brutal talons of the pelican and the key. An advertisement in the *Daily Courant* of 30 December 1717 claimed of a powder:[1]

> It at once makes the teeth as white as ivory, tho' never so black or yellow, and effectually preserves them from rotting or decaying, continuing them sound to exceeding old age. It wonderfully cures the scurvy in the gums, prevents rheum or defluxions, kills worms at the root of the teeth, and thereby hinders the tooth-ach. It admirably fastens loose teeth, being a neat and cleanly medicine of a pleasant and graceful scent.

An even more ridiculous claim is made just over a hundred years later in an advertisement on the front page of *The Times* for 15 August 1821, and illustrates how little dentistry had progressed from the early eighteenth to the early nineteenth century:

> A Discovery has lately been introduced which bids fair to supersede the necessity of a dentist. Hudson's Botanic Tooth Powder is a certain remedy and preventative for all disorders of the Mouth. It not only cleans and beautifies the Teeth, but preserves them from decay to the latest period of life. It makes them white, fastens such as are loose, prevents those decayed from growing worse, removes the tartar, and cures the scurvy in the gums, leaving them firm and of a healthy redness. It is an antidote for

[1] Menzies Campbell.

gum-boils, swelled face, and that excruciating pain called tooth-ache; and so certain and undeviating in its effects, that there never was an instance of any person who used it ever having the tooth-ache or tooth decay; and though so efficacious an antiseptic, it is so innocent that the contents of a box may be swallowed by an infant without any danger.

This multi-purpose tooth-powder was sold by Gatti and Pearce, 57 New Bond Street, London, and by Mr Atkinson, 44 Gerrard Street. It must have seemed well worth a try at a shilling or so the box. One tincture for preparing at home was a mixture of honey, myrrh, juniper root and rock alum; another, roasted turnip parings for putting behind the ear.

On finding such preparations useless for their aches, many people, of course, just let rotting teeth die slowly in the mouth as they crumbled away. Advertisements for false teeth worked in phrases like 'no extraction of stumps' and 'can be worn over the most tender roots or gums'. Here is a typical one – from the *Daily Telegraph* of 2 April 1866:

> Mr Day, 291 Regent Street, London, for many years principal assistant to Mr Eskell, Surgeon-Dentist: Artificial teeth, exquisitely enamelled to nature, made and fitted (in a few hours if required) without extraction of roots of teeth, or giving any pain whatever. Discoloured teeth restored, loose teeth fastened. . . .

There was no deception about the initial whitening effect of tooth-powders made from coral or pumice. Nearly all were so gritty they wore away tooth enamel as well as stains (though not as fast as the caustics often used). For application at home, lemon juice mixed with burnt alum and salt was recommended. Berdmore, experimenting with a usual brand of powder on a drawn tooth held in a vice, found that half an hour's continuous rubbing was enough to take off the enamel entirely.

Intelligent people who believed they had found an effective yet not too abrasive tooth-powder were inclined, in the phrase of a modern paste advertisement, to swear by it. In a letter to the Prince Regent, Prince Ernest once wrote:

> P.S. I have a favor to beg of you; do when you come bring me some of Dumergue's tooth-powder.[1]

[1] *The Correspondence of George Prince of Wales.* Ed. A. Aspinal.

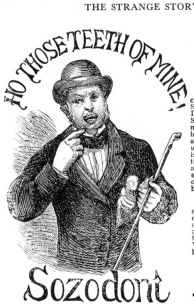

H⁰! THOSE ᴛEETH OF Mᴵᴺᴱ!

—

SOZODONT preserves the Teeth, SOZODONT cleanses the Teeth, SOZODONT beautifies the Teeth, SOZODONT imparts the most fragrant breath, SOZODONT removes all tartar and scurf from the Teeth, SOZODONT arrests the progress of decay. All blemishes that disfigure the Teeth are speedily removed by SOZODONT, the great purifying and beautifying agent. The gums are made rosy and healthy by its use, and the mortifying defect, an unpleasant breath, is completely remedied by it. It is the king of dentifrices. The bottles are fitted with patent sprinklers for applying the liquid to the toothbrush. Each bottle is enclosed in a toilet box. Ask for SOZODONT, and observe the name SOZODONT on the label, box, and bottle.

The daily demand for SOZODONT is a marvel in the annals of toilet requisites. It exceeds that of all other dentifrices combined. This famous article is one of acknowledged merit, and those who once use it will always use it; hence its immense sale.—It is supplied by all Chemists and Perfumers, or direct from the Wholesale Agent (a single bottle at 3s. 6d., or 4 bottles for 10s).

—

Jᴏʜɴ M. RICHARDS,
GREAT RUSSELL STREET, LONDON.

Advertisement for a probably dangerous tooth-whitener. 1880.

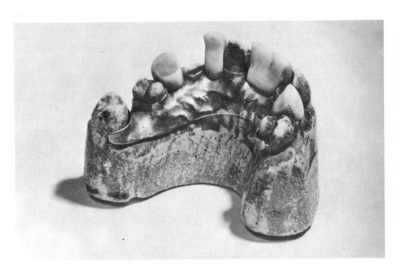

Gold upper plate with carved ivory teeth made for William Duke of Clarence (later William IV) by Isaac Wilson of Bath. Teeth shown on the original plaster cast of the jaw.

44

Charles Dumergue, a naturalized British subject, was an operator for the teeth often patronized by both the Prince Regent and his mother.

As tools for home teeth-cleansing, cloths and sponges were still thought adequate. Brushes were rarities, or at any rate luxuries, till after about 1850. The well-to-do kept quill or metal toothpicks about their persons (as in Roman times); there were also handsome sets of scalers for gentlemen to have among their articles of the toilet.

In Paris the wiser practice of using bits of wood seems to have been more prevalent. Jean Renoir writes that his grandparents in the first half of the nineteenth century 'washed out their mouths, night and morning, with salt water and cleaned their teeth with little wooden tooth-picks, which were then thrown away'.[1]

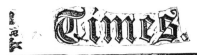

1821.   PRICE 7d.

SUPERIOR Shawls.—Witham and Sons are now introducing a great variety of their new patterns in long and square Shawls, which will be found very superior to any hitherto introduced, as well as considerably under the usual prices. They are also receiving a succession of novelties in Fashionable Morning and Evening Dresses, Fancy Scarfs, &c.—104, Fleet Street, corner of New Bridge Street.

COALS, 40s.; Best Wallsend, 44s. per Chaldron, for ready money, delivered on the stones, except shooting and metage, with three sacks in grain in five Chaldrons, delivered by the Pelican Sea Coal Company. Families who are in want of a good article and measure, may depend upon the above Company. A line to their agents will be punctually attended to.
Mr. Wakefield, 2, Lamb's Conduit Street; Mr. Scrooley, bootmaker, 165, Oxford Street; Mr. Reed, 55, Charing Cross; and Mr. Stephenson, 102, Holborn Hill, corner of Ely Place.

PATENT Reverting Spring Trusses.—Lodge and Bittlestone, 128, Strand, having obtained the King's Letters Patent for Trusses of an entirely new construction, which obviates the great evil arising from the pressure of the spring upon the back, and which are approved and recommended for the relief of Hernia by the most eminent Surgeons, beg leave to inform the public that they are to be had in London only of the Patentees as above, and of William Sheldrake, 483, Strand.
N.B.—Persons residing in those country towns where the Patentees have not yet appointed agents, on sending their measure round the hips, may rely on being accurately fitted.

EASE and Economy in Shaving.—To those

CHAMPAGNE.—DALE, 27, Coventry Street, has the honour to inform Families that the above Wine (well up) is in the highest state of perfection; warranted four years old; manufactured from the finest grapes, and of superior flavour to most of the Champagne imported, and charged from seven to nine guineas per dozen. Price of the article 36s. per dozen; single bottles for sample, 3s. 6d. Country orders per remittance, one dozen, £2; half dozen, £1, hamper and bottles included.

A Discovery has lately been introduced which bids fair to supersede the necessity of a Dentist. Hudson's Botanic Tooth Powder is a certain remedy and preventative for all the disorders of the Mouth. It not only cleanses and beautifies the Teeth, but preserves them from decay to the latest period of life. It makes them white, fastens such as are loose, prevents those decayed growing worse, removes the tartar, and curds the scurvy in the gums, leaving them firm, and of a healthy redness. It is an antidote for gum-boils, swelled face, and that excruciating pain called tooth-ache; and so certain and undeviating in its effects, that there never was an instance of any person who used it ever having the tooth-ache or a tooth decay; and though so efficacious an antiseptic, it is so innocent that the contents of a box may be swallowed by an infant without any danger.
The following agents are appointed:—Mr. Atkinson, 44, Gerard Street; Sanger, 150, Oxford Street; Gatti and Pearce, 57, New Bond Street; and most perfumers.

WANTED, a respectable Servant of All Work, about 30 years of age, where a Nursemaid is kept; one from the country would be pre-

[1] J. Renoir, *My Father*, 1958.

45

7

French False Teeth

The first effective method of attaching an upper set of teeth to a toothless jaw – that is, by metal springs fixed to the lower set – was developed by Pierre Fauchard (1678–1761), a Parisian surgeon and practising dentist who probably did more than anyone to help make dentistry a profession instead of a trade. His treatise *Le Chirurgien Dentiste*, 1728, includes detailed information and drawings to do with the making of false teeth. Fauchard was unusual in seeking to guide others at a time when even reputable practitioners were inclined to keep quiet about their methods for fear of competition.

There was no prejudice against false teeth among the large well-to-do society of eighteenth-century Paris, whose passion for elegance took in details of personal appearance. Gaps in front were not only disfiguring, they also interfered with dignified speech. 'Without teeth,' said a Parisian *dentiste* (the word now used in France), 'some people cannot make any distinct and perfectly articulated sound, and it often happens that what they wish to express cannot be comprehended.' So missing teeth had at all costs to be replaced; the carvers of ivory ornaments became the first dental mechanics. Although, in the words of a contemporary observer, the replacements looked like the keyboard of a spinet, they were preferable in *salon* circles to bare gums.

Parisians lacking upper teeth suitable for anchorage would even submit to the horrifying expedient of having the gums pierced to allow a row of teeth, fitted with two hooks, to be suspended from them on the ear-ring principle. 'Floating teeth', Fauchard observed, 'obeying every impulse of the tongue and of the air entering and leaving the mouth'. A sensitive man, he was genuinely upset over the way such pieces dragged and worried the gums:

> I heard of one lady so equipped who had nothing but torment until a happy fit of coughing sent the troublesome denture into the fire. . . . The lady must indeed have had a great desire to have her mouth supplied to endure such a cruel operation, and at the same time such a ridiculous one, without a thought for the dangerous consequences that might arise. I cannot conceive how a dentist who has any regard for his reputation should expose a person thus, especially in Paris, where so many good dentists practise – and contribute by their work to the ornament of this beautiful town.

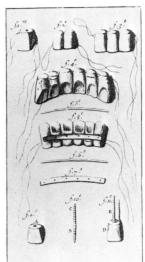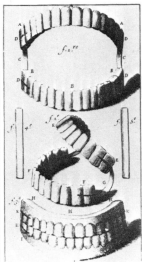

LEFT: *Crowns and bridges by Fauchard. From his book* Le Chirugien Dentiste, 1728.

RIGHT: *His full sets: fig. 3 shows an enamelled set with gums, fig. 4 and fig. 5 steel springs.*

Fauchard's retention springs of flat steel (an improvement on slips of whalebone which had been tried) had their ends fastened at the back of the upper and lower denture. Once in the mouth, they exerted a constant pressure which forced the artificial teeth into contact with the gums. Naturally some muscular effort was needed to shut the mouth – which partially opened in repose – but at least top sets with these powerful stabilizers never fell.

Patients who had lost only their top teeth, and had thus no lower dentures to which springs could be hinged, presented a problem. Fauchard writes as follows in a revised edition of his book:

> In 1737 a lady of high rank, about the age of sixty, who had not lost any of her lower teeth but was deprived entirely of the upper ones, applied to M. Caperon, dentist to the King and a man most able in his profession, in the hope that he might be able to furnish her mouth with an upper set. But he said that, no tooth whatever being left, every possible point of attachment was wanting and it would therefore be as difficult to do this as to build in the air.

The lady then went to see Fauchard in the Rue de la Comédie Française, and explained to him that all she wanted was to pronounce better and have the front of her mouth decorated. Fauchard asked for a few days to think the matter

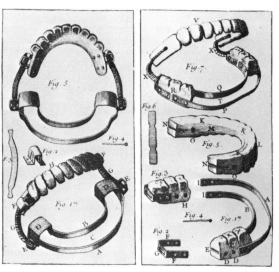

Fauchard appliances for mouths where at least some of the lower teeth survive.

over. In due course he produced an abbreviated type of upper set, embellished by his enameller, which was supported by a framework on the lower teeth and gums.

Apparently she was well satisfied with the appliance. Writing a few years afterwards, Fauchard reports with a hint of surprise that she ate with it. 'She could not now do without it and for greater convenience she has two similar sets which she uses alternately.'

Fauchard offers encouragement to beginners:

> Let not the use of things unfamiliar to us, and which at first appear strange, discourage us. The inconvenience of the first few days is only transitory and a circumstance necessarily associated with a fault in use – that is, if the discomfort is not the fault of an incapable artist, who may have been clumsy in the making of the pieces not having observed all the details I have exactly recorded.

Although an upper set on springs gave its wearer confidence in talk and laughter, skilled control by the cheeks was needed for any kind of chewing, since there was little to stop it slipping painfully from one side to the other. A plate covering the whole palate (not yet thought of) and a U-shaped rim of artificial gum would have checked the lateral movement, but bulk was avoided to ease the task of inserting both sets in the mouth together.

Because of abominable discomfort at meals, people with full sets, or dentures that were not tied in, would often take them out on coming to the table, the men putting them back later to help their enunciation over the port. This, incidentally, was chemically unfortunate in view of port's darkening effect on ivory – as a dentist once explained to George Washington.

Around the middle of the eighteenth century the flat, back-fastening springs, which could irritate the throat, began to be dropped in favour of coil springs fastened at the sides of the sets in the region of the first molars above and below. These were found to spread the pressure more evenly over the jaws and to lessen a tendency for the lower set to strain forward and push out the lip. Berdmore called them 'springs of a new and peculiar

construction' which were gentle in their action. Sets of teeth
fitted with them

> answer every purpose of the natural Teeth and can be taken out,
> cleaned, and replaced by the patient himself, with the greatest
> ease.

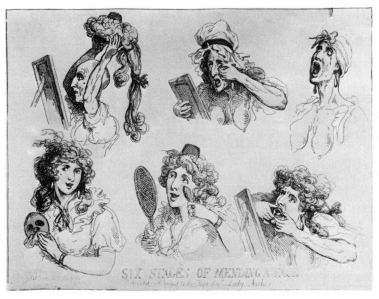

Rowlandson's Six Stages of Mending a Face *(1792) – to be viewed from right
to left. Elderly ladies of fashion were often ridiculed by eighteenth-century carica-
turists. Lady Archer (1741–1801), widow of the 2nd Baron Archer, was a noted
whip and noted also for over-painting her face. In* Miscellaneous Poetry *Lord
Townshend referred to 'Lacker faced A-ch-r'. Horace Walpole remarked in a letter
'A was an Archer and painted her face'. Note the hare's foot for applying rouge
(bottom centre) and the mask held in the hand (bottom left).*

In the latter part of the century a wax more or less suitable
for taking mouth impressions was evolved. Philip Pfaff, dentist
to Frederick the Great of Prussia, is believed to have been the
first to make plaster casts of an entire jaw from wax impressions. To avoid distorting the wax on removing it from the
mouth, he is said to have taken an impression first of one side
then the other and joined the two together.[1]

[1] Guerini.

8

The All-porcelain Set

Herrick was wrong in writing that teeth of bone would not rot. As organic, porous materials, bone and ivory normally began to blacken and decay within a year from the action of oral fluids. The weakness was emphasized in an early Victorian handbook on the use and management of artificial teeth:[1]

> It is of great importance that you should know how to preserve false teeth, for in the absence of proper attention they are soon destroyed, and still sooner become offensive. The wearer often seems singularly unconscious of the offensive odour which arises from neglected teeth – not so, however, the bystander; he is almost poisoned by the offensive breath of his neighbour . . . dentine [ivory], when highly polished, resists the action of the saliva, and therefore is not subject to decomposition. The wearer should pay great attention to this point. The surfaces of the teeth . . . should be well brushed with a little precipitated chalk, once or twice a day; and after brushing, rubbed with a dry soft towel. . . .

In the 1790s there had been news of false teeth with base and teeth made in one solid piece of shiny, rot-proof porcelain. These were the once-celebrated de Chemant mineral-paste dentures for which Nicholas Dubois de Chemant, a Paris-trained dentist, had no difficulty in obtaining testimonials. Edward Jenner, discoverer of vaccination, wrote one; so did Monsieur Geoffroy, President of the Royal Society of Medicine in Paris:

> I declare that the success is superior to my hopes. I further attest, that the teeth of sea horse which I wore for only one year, had so

[1] John Tomes, *The Management of Artificial Teeth*, 1851.

51

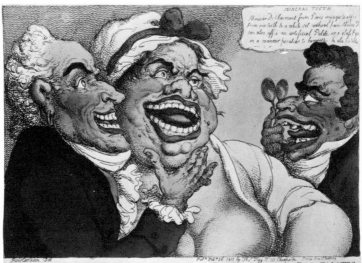

A Rowlandson print (1811) of the French dentist, Dubois de Chemant, showing off the mouth of a woman fitted with a double row of his mineral paste teeth and gums. So wide is her smile, the springs between them can just be seen. A man in great need of dental treatment stares through a double lorgnette. By 1811 full sets of mineral paste were beginning to fall into disrepute.

much disgusted me, by the bad smell they gave to my breath, and the disagreeable taste they communicated to my food, that I had not only withdrawn myself from company, but taken them out to eat.

I no longer doubt, Sir, that my ill state of health proceeded from the putrid miasma given out by the bony substance of this set of teeth . . . since I have laid it aside, and have used yours, my health is infinitely improved. I eat with more facility. . . .

By your discovery, you have without doubt rendered a service to humanity; let us hope, that soon private gatherings and public places will no longer be infected by those animal substances . . . imagine two thousand people at the opera, there may be amongst them, at least, two or three hundred who have a small piece of sea horse tooth in the mouth; form an idea of all those decayed substances, and you will have a skeleton of the animal, which, if placed on the stage, would soon drive away all the spectators by the putrefaction and disgust it would occasion.

SEA HORSE TEETH,

THE DENTIST has received in addition, a new for the purpose of making artificial Teeth, which he intends for the use of his practice, the enamel of which is much thicker than the human teeth, and so hard as to produce fire equal to a flint, and so nigh the colour, that when formed into the shape of human teeth, they cannot be perceived from them by the most strict observer. He makes whole sets of teeth, and fixes them in the mouth where there is neither tooth nor stump, they are fixed with springs in such a manner as to permit the teeth to act with every motion of the jaw, both horizontal and perpendicular, without causing the least pain or uncleanness, being useful in every point as other teeth; the springs are fixed in, so as neither to be seen nor felt. Those who would wish to have them fix'd, may be better informed by their humble servant the Dentist, whose practice is universally approved of, and who will exert his utmost abilities to heal every deficiency, so as to render your teeth the most brilliant ornaments that can be exposed to view.

N. B. He cures the Scurvy, and ulcerated gums, and by your observance of his directions, the Scurvy will never return.

Transplants and grafts natural Teeth. A generous price given for Teeth, either dead or alive, by   J. GREENWOOD,

Oct. 4.   *Surgeon Dentist,*

No. 56, William-street, corner of Beekman Street.

From the American Daily Advertiser, *October 15, 1790. Sea horse means walrus tusk.*

The true originator of the new type of denture was not de Chemant but a French apothecary, Alexis Duchâteau of St-Germain-en-Laye, near Paris. He had been wearing for some years a set made of hippopotamus ivory which had grown especially disagreeable to him – tainting all he ate – because of the chemical preparations he had to taste in his work. The teeth had also become stained, so it is said, with splashes of colour – red, blue and green predominating; even with an array of

E   53

chemicals at his disposal, he could find nothing that would bleach the colours away.

The constant annoyance and embarrassment gave him the idea of having his denture reproduced in porcelain. He applied to a china factory. The first trial was a complete failure: the porcelain shrank so much under firing that the result was unwearable. Trying to allow for this, he had the potters start with an out-size model; it contracted to the wrong size.

There were numerous trials before a set was produced which Duchâteau judged fit to wear. But as it seemed grotesquely white, he had it given a yellow tint. Unfortunately the second baking needed for fixing the colour distorted the porcelain once more and he could not get the teeth in his mouth.

Putting them aside, Duchâteau began a new series of experiments with a special kind of porcelain paste which vitrified at a lower temperature. There were more near misses. Eventually he sought the help of a dentist, and picked on de Chemant. Together they modified the paste, adding pipeclay and colouring earths, and found they could bake it at a still lower temperature. Eventually they turned out a denture which fitted Duchâteau's gums reasonably well and which, in fact, he proceeded to wear in daily life.

Much encouraged, he tried to make money by supplying similar sets for others; but he lacked dental knowledge and grotesquely failed. In 1776 he laid the new process before the Royal Academy of Surgeons in Paris and was rewarded by their thanks and an honourable mention. He did no more.

De Chemant, on the other hand, never ceased from working at the invention. He determined to calculate exactly the degree to which china teeth would contract on heating, and to perfect the system of springs for holding them in place. He persevered to good effect: there were several people wearing the new sort of teeth when in 1788 he published a book on them.[1]

In this he lashed out at the use of ivory, bone and other animal substances, and drew attention to the incorruptible and therefore healthy nature of his mineral paste. His case histories

[1] Dubois de Chemant, *A Dissertation on Artificial Teeth*, Paris, 1797.

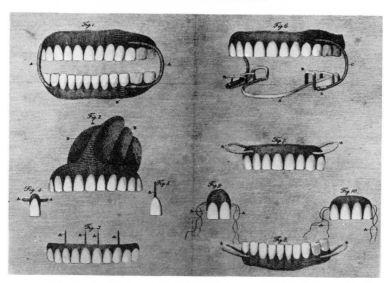

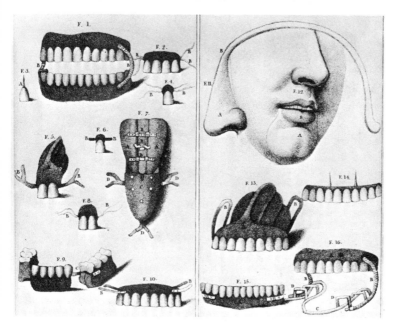

Mineral paste teeth and obturators by de Chemant, showing methods of attachment. From A Dissertation on Artificial Teeth, *1802.*

55

– though possibly exaggerated with a view to advertisement – open the eyes to a form of dental suffering little considered today:

> Having been called in to examine the mouth of a lady of quality, who felt herself gradually declining in a slow fever . . . I found that the artificial teeth of animal substance which she had, were become black, and exhaled a fetid and unsupportable smell. . . . I did not hesitate to declare that the fever was occasioned and continued by the absorption of the infected matter which came off the rotten teeth. . . . They were removed [most likely they were semi-permanently wired in place] and the fever ceased in a few days.

M. Geoffroy in 1790 sent him one of his patients,

> seventy years old, burdensome to himself and to all who came near him, on account of the stench of his breath. I remarked that he had a complete set of *human teeth* mounted on an *ivory base*. After having removed this cause of infection and sickness, I made him a complete set of teeth of mineral paste, and had the satisfaction to see him recover his health in a short time.

De Chemant prospered. The Paris Faculty of Medicine pronounced that his dentures 'united the qualities of beauty, solidity and comfort to the exigencies of hygiene'; King Louis XVI granted him an inventor's patent and Général Comte de Martagne, aged eighty-two, wrote a poem:

> When time has stripped our armoury bare,
> Dubois steps in with subtle heed;
> New grinders and new cutters gives;
> With his we laugh, with his we feed.
> Long live Chemant, friend in need.

The publicity upset other Parisian dentists, who found a way to bring an action against de Chemant by accusing him of having stolen Duchâteau's invention: de Chemant had claimed full credit for his process, saying in so many words that the idea had been entirely his own. Although the action failed, de Chemant decided to move – the French Revolution was

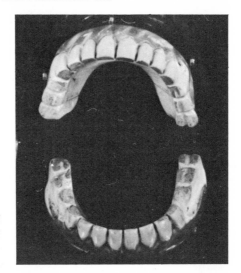

De Chemant all-porcelain full upper and lower set with biting surfaces grown rough from use. c. 1800.

beginning to affect his practice; and he emigrated, as some of his best patients were doing, to England.

He set up in London in 1792, there securing without difficulty the exclusive right, for fourteen years, of manufacturing dentures of porcelain paste (the Wedgwood factory supplied it). He claimed that by 1804 there were 12,000 of his dentures in use.

For extra strength, the teeth were not separated along their length, merely shaded. Although immediately striking the eye as art work, they and their pink porcelain gums at least looked

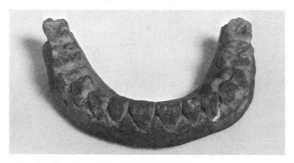

A badly chipped and discoloured lower denture in porcelain which was probably never glazed. Early nineteenth century.

shiny and fresh. Naturally the grinding surfaces lost their glaze after a time, enabling a jealous London dentist[1] to deride these 'boasted teeth of a foreigner' as 'nothing more or less than earthenwear'. There were unfortunate cases of cracking in half, sometimes in the mouth. But what really brought the craze to an end was the inability of de Chemant's imitators to make them fit properly. He had plenty of imitators, all anxious to be up to date, but some so unskilled in porcelain work that patients were made grotesque by their appliances.

However, dentists continued to be fascinated by the idea. As late as 1854 full dentures made entirely of porcelain were re-introduced by the American dentist Mahlon Loomis, who patented his process in America, England and France. There was also a Luxembourg pastry cook who thought of porcelain independently and made a successful denture in 1862.[2] William Dunn of Cleveland, Ohio, took out a patent in 1867 on a method which was actually almost identical with that of de Chemant. However, except for making bases to fill small gaps, the all-porcelain construction never attained importance.

---

[1] T. M. Patence, Strand, London – Menzies Campbell.
[2] *Revue d'histoire de l'art dentaire*, No 3.

9

Waterloo Teeth

Although de Chemant's mineral paste could not after all fulfil a dream, its freedom from decay did stimulate work on individual teeth made of porcelain for attaching to plates of ivory or metal. Teeth of this variety, greatly improved, are to this day supreme: the modern acrylic resin teeth, on pleasant-looking bases of the same material, are easy to make life-like but have the disadvantage of softness and gradually wearing away.

The first single porcelain teeth were launched in 1808 by an Italian dentist, Guiseppangelo Fonzi, who worked in Paris. They became known as bean teeth because the front ones closely resembled a split bean: they were rounded, enamelled on the outside and perfectly flat on the inside. For mounting on denture bases, small metal hooks or loops were embedded in the porcelain.

There was immediate interest in dental circles in England. Bartholomew Ruspini, a surgeon-dentist to the fashionable in London and Bath, was one of the first to hear of them. A conversation over dinner at his house is described in a letter of August 1808, signed F. Hall, to the painter John Vanderlyn, who knew Fonzi in Paris:[1]

Being at dinner the other day, with Chevalier Ruspini, Surgeon-Dentist to the Prince of Wales, and not a little occupied in masticating a fine haunch of roasted beef, teeth became the subject of conversation. Several kinds of artificial grinders were, of course, mentioned, and, among others, I took an opportunity to notice those with which your friend is now ornamenting the jaw

[1] *Squibbs Memoranda*, New York, 1931.

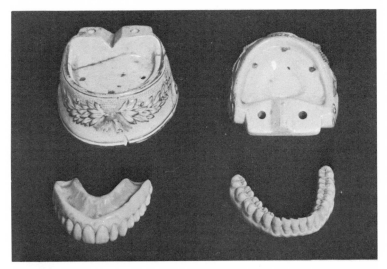

Display holder, attributed to Ruspini, and teeth before being assembled.

bones of the Parisians. This excited the curiosity of the Chevalier, who earnestly solicited me to assist him in getting a peep at his brother Italian's late celebrated discovery; and promising, that if he could approve of it, after examination, he would employ his utmost exertions to be of service to the author in England. He wished not only for a tooth or two, but to be informed of the manner in which they were fastened in.

However, the so-called mineral teeth long remained imperfect, despite numerous experiments in France, which exported them. They had a very artificial appearance in the mouth and made a grating sound when brought together. They

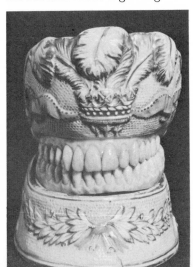

Ivory dentures on so-called Ruspini display holder (decorated with Prince of Wales feathers motif). c. 1805.

60

were over-white, opaque and brittle. Nearly forty years after their introduction, a dentist of standing wrote as follows:

> The things called mineral, or Jews' teeth, are now plentifully manufactured of porcelain; but they always look like what they are, and can never be mistaken for teeth . . . and by acting as a whetstone on any of the natural teeth . . . soon wear them away.[1]

For all its disadvantages, ivory was not quickly ousted as the normal material for artificial teeth and the bases for them. A nineteenth-century recipe for Ivory Dust Jelly, by Emma Gurney, suggested a way of using up a plentiful by-product:

> Boil a pound of Ivory dust in a gallon of water until the liquid is reduced to one half. Strain it through a jelly bag, and when cold make the same use of it as the stock of calf's foot.

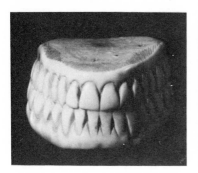 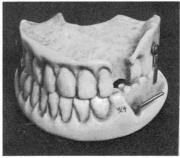

LEFT: *Late eighteenth-century ivory advertisement piece.*

RIGHT: *As it might have been worked up for a customer with fittings for slipping on spiral retention springs.*

The firm of Claudius Ash, London, were supplying ivory blocks for denture work as recently as 1875.

The demand continued, too, for human teeth plundered from the corpses of vault and battlefield by characters known as resurrectionists. These could sometimes deceive the eye provided they were kept steady on the gums and slightly covered by the lips.

Even when a corpse was badly decomposed, its front teeth

[1] John Gray, *Preservation of the Teeth*, 1838.

remained saleable. There are accounts of nineteenth-century resurrectionists realizing £20 to £30 for the teeth found in a single vault. 'Oh, Sir, only let there be a battle and there'll be no want of teeth,' says a character in B.B. Cooper's *Life of Sir Astley Paston Cooper*. 'I'll draw them as fast as the men are knocked down!'

Many people unknowingly wore teeth extracted from young men on the field of Waterloo. The label Waterloo teeth is not a contemporary one. Gruesome and downright unhygienic as the use of such objects now seems, it may be surmised that in the

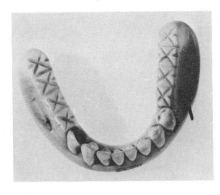

Ivory lower piece fitted with human front teeth which may well have come from the field of Waterloo. The teeth of healthy young men were in great demand and battles offered a useful supply. c. 1820.

twenty-first century it will be thought equally unpleasant that the best wigs and toupees of the 1960s were made of human hair.

Almost certainly the re-used teeth sometimes brought infection. They were subject to decay in the mouth, though to a slightly less extent than the porous ivory teeth. Disinfectants had not been thought of in these times, but at least there is evidence of human teeth having been boiled before delivery to the patient.

They were used less in the second half of the nineteenth century, though they remained on offer to dentists, and were still considered an ordinary article of commerce. They appear, in various grades, in the 1862 catalogue of Smale Brothers, dental suppliers. In 1865 the *Pall Mall Gazette* observed that certain dentists in London did not trouble to make artificial teeth; instead they used natural ones collected from the battlefields of the American Civil War by a horde of tooth-drawers who followed the armies. (They were, in truth, shipped to England by the barrel.[1])

From about 1845 dentists were all the same making increasing use of an improved type of ready-made porcelain tooth on sale to them – a much better article than most dentists could make for themselves. The rich might be charged up to 150 guineas for a single set of 'incorrodible mineral teeth'. In an attempt to help the poor, the young ladies of at least one Victorian family are known to have devoted several afternoons a week to the modelling of individual artificial teeth.

Samuel Stockton of Philadelphia, his nephew S. S. White, and Claudius Ash – founder of the firm still bearing his name – contributed greatly to improvements in the commercial article. Ash, a silversmith at the beginning of the nineteenth century, became interested in teeth when a London dentist asked him to reproduce a dental appliance. He did the job so skilfully that he soon found himself spending most of his time on work for dentists. He became one of the first dental mechanics.[2]

Most of his work was riveting human teeth to ivory bases, each set taking him about six weeks. But he disliked handling dead men's teeth and began experiments with porcelain in the hope of improving on the French bean teeth. He succeeded, and in due course was able to embark on large-scale manufacture of porcelain teeth in several shades of light grey. In dental circles today, modern Ash teeth are famous.

They are of course no longer grey. Greyness and the tell-tale chinawear appearance became unnecessary at the end of the 1930s. One of the first to achieve a semi-translucent, slightly orange tooth was Dr Simon Myerson of Massachusetts. In 1940 he demonstrated a set in the mouth of an elderly colleague at the Waldorf–Astoria Hotel, Manhattan. 'See,' he cried, 'how becoming they are to the rugged character time has produced in his face.' Whereupon, according to a *Time* report of the event, all present rose as one man and applauded the teeth.

[1] Menzies Campbell.   [2] M. D. K. Bremner, *The Story of Dentistry*, 1954.

10

Springs

Whatever the materials used for teeth and bases, gold coil springs long continued a standard holding-in device. In *King Solomon's Mines* by Rider Haggard (1885) Captain Good's nervous habit of plucking at his top set electrifies a savage tribe which he and his companions encounter in Africa.

'What does the beggar say?' asked Good.

'He says we are going to be killed,' I answered grimly.

'Oh, Lord!' groaned Good; and, as was his way when perplexed, he put his hand to his false teeth, dragging the top set down and allowing them to fly back to his jaw with a snap. It was a most fortunate move, for next second the dignified crowd of Kukuanas uttered a simultaneous yell of horror, and bolted back some yards.

'What's up?' said I.

'It's his teeth,' whispered Sir Henry excitedly. 'He moved them. Take them out, Good, take them out!'

He obeyed, slipping the set into the sleeve of his flannel shirt.

In another second curiosity had overcome fear, and the men advanced slowly. Apparently they had now forgotten their amiable intention of killing us.

'How is it, O strangers,' asked the old man solemnly, 'that this fat man . . . has teeth which move of themselves, coming away from the jaws and returning of their own free will?'

'Open your mouth,' I said to Good, who promptly curled up his lips and grinned at the old gentleman like an angry dog, revealing to his astonished gaze two thin lines of gum as utterly innocent of ivories as is a new-born elephant. The audience gasped.

'Where are his teeth?' they shouted; 'with our eyes we saw them.'

Turning his head slowly and with a gesture of ineffable con-
tempt, Good swept his hand across his mouth. Then he grinned
again, and lo, there were two rows of lovely teeth.

The old man's knees knocked together with fear. 'I see that ye
are spirits,' he said falteringly; 'did ever man born of woman have
. . . teeth which moved and melted away and grew again? Pardon
us, O my lords.'

Clearly Captain Good was neat fingered. In the hands of the
less experienced, it was all too easy for false-teeth springs to get
in a tangle or come adrift. John Tomes, a surgeon-dentist to the
Middlesex Hospital, gives detailed advice in his little book,
The Management of Artificial Teeth (1851):

> Teeth retained by spiral springs require considerable care in
> putting them into the mouth. The wearer not infrequently injures
> or entirely destroys 2 or 3 pairs of springs by bad management,
> before experience has taught the manner of avoiding such
> accidents. The proper position of the springs when the teeth are
> in, and the mouth closed, is shown in fig. 5, and any deviation
> from that position will be attended with injury to the apparatus.

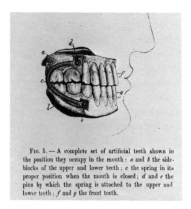

Fig. 5. — A complete set of artificial teeth shown in
the position they occupy in the mouth : *a* and *b* the side-
blocks of the upper and lower teeth ; *c* the spring in its
proper position when the mouth is closed ; *d* and *e* the
pins by which the spring is attached to the upper and
lower teeth ; *f* and *g* the front teeth.

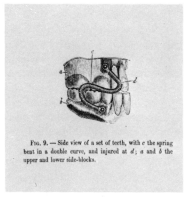

Fig. 9. — Side view of a set of teeth, with *c* the spring
bent in a double curve, and injured at *d* ; *a* and *b* the
upper and lower side-blocks.

If, for instance, a spring should get into the position shown at
fig. 9, it will be so damaged, if not absolutely broken, that its
action will ever after be imperfect; or if it should be allowed to
project forwards towards the lips, great inconvenience will be felt,
and the spring, if not speedily released, will most likely be
permanently injured.

Springs' failures could be worse than inconvenient, since

without their aid few top sets would hold up even in conversation. Disaster was at hand for the Victorian lady caught without a second pair. Tomes goes on to give explicit instructions on how to avoid 'unpleasant accidents'.

In one method the upper and lower teeth should be placed with the masticating surfaces in contact, and with the springs in the position shown in fig. 5; the forefingers should then be placed over the upper, and the thumbs under the lower teeth. In this manner the upper and lower teeth can be held firmly together: when so held, one side should be passed a short distance within the lips and with it the cheeks pressed outwards. By this means the mouth will be stretched sufficiently open to allow the other side of the teeth to be introduced without any fear of the spring becoming entangled with the lips, which, but for this precaution, would probably pass in between the spring and the teeth.

Having once got the teeth fairly into the mouth, they will almost of themselves find their proper position on the gums. However, it is desirable to press the base well into its place before attempting to close the mouth.

The second method . . . is effected in the following manner. Instead of placing the upper and lower teeth in the mouth together, the 2 parts of the set may be put in one after the other.

The upper part of the set may be first pressed lightly into its place and held there by the help of the tongue. The lower division will then project from the mouth, and the springs connecting the two will remain straight, or nearly so. The second step of the process – that of placing the lower teeth – needs some little care, or the springs will suffer more or less injury in the operation. The forefingers should be placed on the masticating surface of the teeth, in doing which the springs will be passed a little backwards, so as to make a backward curve, extending through the whole length of the spring, and similar in direction, though less in degree, to that which they assume when the teeth are properly placed in the mouth. Having grasped the lower teeth, and got the springs in the proper position, in the manner described and shown in fig. 10, they may, without difficulty, be pressed into the mouth.

In some sets it will be found more convenient to place the lower teeth in the mouth first. In such a case the upper ones should be held in the left hand, while with the right the lower teeth are laid upon the gums. Having done this, the thumbs should be placed on the masticating surface of the upper teeth, in which act the springs

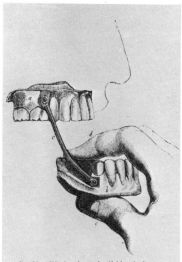

FIG. 10.—Side view of a set of artificial teeth, showing the manner of putting them into the mouth : *a* the upper teeth placed in the mouth with the spring, *c* projecting forward ; *b* the lower teeth, with the forefinger, *d*, placed on the masticating surface, and bending the spring slightly backwards, *e* the thumb.

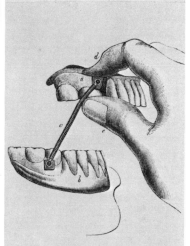

FIG. 11.—Side view of set of teeth, showing the manner of putting them into the mouth when the lower teeth are first placed : *b* the lower teeth already placed in the mouth ; *c* the spring projecting forwards and upwards ; *a* the upper teeth ; *d* the forefinger ; *e* the thumb placed on the masticating surface, so that in pressing the upper teeth into the mouth, the spring will assume its proper position.

at their middle part should be pressed backwards towards the mouth, in the same manner as I have described when speaking of the lower teeth, when they are the last to be introduced. The springs being grasped in the manner shown in fig. 11, and the springs bent backwards in a single curve, they will readily pass into the mouth. . . .

A spring which has once been permanently bent can never be restored to its former condition, and from that time will act but imperfectly . . . springs, however carefully manufactured and used, will sometimes break suddenly and without any obvious cause . . . it is of great consequence the spring should move freely on the swivels, otherwise it will be almost impossible to avoid an accident.

Accidents apart, coil springs had several disadvantages, of which one of the least supportable was the impossibility of throughly cleaning them. Patients complained of a sense of weight and falling in the lower jaw. One mid-nineteenth-century textbook actually stated that springs 'induce a disposition to paralysis of the muscles of the lower jaw'.

67

But few people had any confidence in the sets designed to stay in place without them. There was always a risk. However ill-fitting a person's plate might be, at least with springs he was

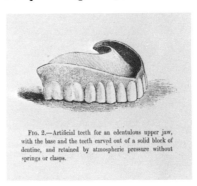

FIG. 2.—Artificial teeth for an edentulous upper jaw, with the base and the teeth carved out of a solid block of dentine, and retained by atmospheric pressure without springs or clasps.

safe in conversation. Springs were economical, too; there was no need to have a new set made simply because of gum shrinkage. Those who had invested in gold rather than ivory bases would keep the same denture for up to forty years; it became an old friend that one could take a pride in being able to manage. There is still, in the 1970s, the occasional elderly person whose teeth are retained with coil springs of stainless steel.

Teeth Without Fastenings

It would be nice to think that a dental mishap of the ultimate kind described below by A.J. Cronin was extremely rare. The passage comes from *Hatter's Castle* (1931), set in the late nineteenth century:

> She broke into peals of shrill laughter, when suddenly, her false teeth, never at any time secure and now dislodged from her palate by her moist exuberance, protruded from between her lips like the teeth of a neighing horse, and impelled by a last uncontrollable spasm of mirth, shot out of her mouth and shattered themselves upon the floor.

Modern top sets are made in such a way that they are readily stabilized by adhesion – the sort which enables a moistened slip of glass to cling to another – and also to some extent by atmospheric pressure or suction. The latter force, which can reach 14 lb, comes into play when all air is driven out from between the base and the parts it rests on; like the force of adhesion, it fails, and the teeth fall down, directly the smallest leak appears at the edge of the plate.

When dislodged in eating, the upwards thrust of the lower jaw should instantly re-establish adhesion and suction. The necessary conditions are a perfect fit everywhere and a plate covering as large an area as the wearer can tolerate.

Adhesion and suction are expected to play a part in the retention of lower dentures, but with these it is nowadays recognized that the base must be splayed out in such a way that the cheek muscles and the back of the tongue instinctively hold it down. The early lower sets, those with neither springs nor

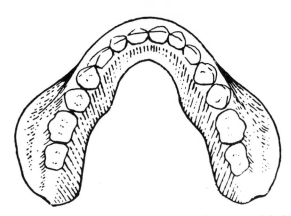

Modern lower denture with base splayed out for tongue and cheek muscles to help hold it down.

anchorage to existing teeth, relied mainly on their weight, which was often made considerable by the inclusion of lead.

Fauchard knew nothing of atmospheric pressure as a means of retention. And since his upper sets were formed in a brief horseshoe shape just like lower ones, there was little opportunity for it to assert itself (plates covering the whole roof of the mouth, as today, were barely even thought of till the 1830s). But Fauchard took infinite care with the fit of his carved ivory bases, and was able to report having three times in his career made upper sets that would stay in place without springs.

In writing of them he admits the need of support from the cheeks and the lower teeth to bring them back into place. His advice to other dentists was to make such sets very light and not to expect them to do much more than improve the appearance and pronunciation. Only a very few people, he said, were able to wear them. Most likely, these few had learned the trick of balancing their false teeth with their tongues.

Forty years after Fauchard's death, a satisfactory springless top set made by James Gardette of Philadelphia was hailed as a dental triumph; he realized why it worked and became established as the discoverer of the use of atmospheric pressure in dentistry. It seems that in the year 1800 he carved a full

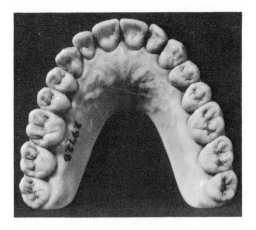

Upper set of carved ivory. Late eighteenth century.

upper set for a woman patient and temporarily left it with her without the springs put on. His son, Emile, kept a record of the sequel:

> It was then still the custom for the dentist to attend at the houses of his patients, and a busy season caused months instead of weeks to elapse, when Mr Gardette called again: with an apology for neglect, his pliers and springs ready, he requested Mrs M'C. to bring the artificial pieces. She replied, 'I have them in my mouth', much to the astonishment of her dentist. . . . She stated that at first they were a little troublesome, but she had become accustomed to them now, and they answered every purpose as well without as with springs, and she was glad to dispense with them. The principle upon which the artificial piece thus adhered to the gums at once suggested itself to his mind, and suction, or atmospheric pressure, was henceforth depended upon in numerous cases of the same kind.

Other dentists were not convinced. B.T. Longbothom, a Londoner who practised in South Carolina, wrote in his *Treatise on Dentistry* (1802):

> Whole sets require springs of a peculiar kind, although once I saw a complete set adhering solely by suction.

(It may have been the one Gardette made for Mrs M'C.) In

71

1848 the United States Patent Office were persuaded that the idea was original (which of course it was not), and granted a patent on false teeth held in place by the pressure of the atmosphere to a Connecticut confectioner.

In England it was not until around 1835 that the notion of suction plates began to be talked about. When occasionally asked for them, dentists did their best to oblige, but often without having much faith in them, or even an understanding of the principle. But that it could ever operate properly with

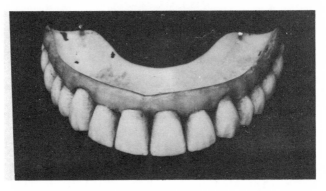

An upper set consisting of a brief ivory base with separately carved ivory teeth attached. Without springs, it was probably extremely unsteady. Early nineteenth century.

upper sets still being made in the traditional horseshoe shape was indeed puzzling.

W. H. Mortimer in his essay on artificial teeth (1845), offered his considered opinion on teeth 'kept in by suction . . . without any fastening whatever':

> I cannot, I confess, understand how they answer. One thing I have invariably observed . . . is that the gums are in a constant state of irritation and inflammation: the tension likewise of the upper lip, to keep them in their place, changes the expression of the face; and as it is a plan that can only now and then succeed, and that only after a long trial, I see no reason for discarding the spiral springs, which always succeed, and in a very short time become quite comfortable.

Painless 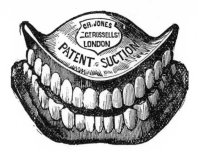 Dentistry.

ARTIFICIAL **TEETH.**

Mr. G. H. JONES, Surgeon Dentist,

57 GREAT RUSSELL STREET, LONDON, W.C.,

(Immediately opposite the British Museum),

Has obtained

HER MAJESTY'S ROYAL LETTERS PATENT

For his improved method of adapting

Artificial Teeth by Atmospheric Pressure.

Note.—Improved Prize Medal Teeth (London and Paris) are adapted in the most difficult and delicate cases, on a perfectly painless system, extraction of loose teeth or stumps being unnecessary, and by recent scientific discoveries and improvements in mechanical dentistry detection is rendered utterly impossible, both by close adjustment of the artificial teeth to the gums and their life-like appearance. By this patented invention complete mastication, extreme lightness, combined with strength and durability, are insured; useless bulk being obviated, articulation is rendered clear and distinct. In the administration of Nitrous Oxide Gas, Mr. G. H. JONES has introduced an entirely new process.

TESTIMONIAL.

My DEAR SIR,—Allow me to express my sincere thanks for the skill and attention displayed in the construction of my Artificial Teeth, which renders my mastication and articulation excellent. I am glad to hear that you have obtained Her Majesty's Royal Letters Patent, to protect what I consider the perfection of Painless Dentistry. In recognition of your valuable services you are at liberty to use my name.

S. G. HUTCHINS,
By appointment Surgeon Dentist to the Queen.

To G. H. JONES, ESQ.

PAMPHLET GRATIS AND POST-FREE.

An advertisement of the 1880s.

73

In the 1860s and 1870s false-teeth advertisements in the newspapers still proclaimed atmospheric pressure as a marvellous new dental invention: 'No springs,' they cried, 'or any other fastening required.' Fastidious patients often found it an embarrassing invention that worked only sometimes, and failed completely at meals. The actual teeth were often so ill-arranged that even a close-fitting denture was at once dislodged on chewing. A false-teeth advertisement of 1866 claimed no more than *usefulness* in mastication. Instead of resorting to springs as the remedy, it was now the practice to fit either air chambers or rubber suction rings in the roofs of plates. Though

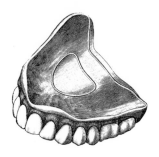

Late nineteenth-century upper set with suction chamber.

reasonably effective, they often injured the mouth, sometimes seriously, by creating intense suction at one point. They have recently been abandoned entirely.

Springs at least did not cause serious injury, but by the end of the century they were supplied with reluctance; dentists saw them as a reflection on their ability to do close-fitting work. Often, however, their plates were failures. Often patients neglected, or could not afford, to go back for adjustments following the normal shrinking of the mouth tissues. Thus began, around 1890, the long era of the dancing top set.

By the 1920s loose appliances of this sort had begun to be described, along with their effect on others, in the con-

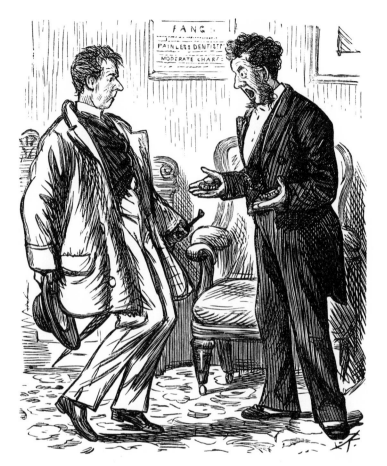

Plain to Demonstration.

Customer (*nervously*). "AH! THEY MUST BE VERY IRKSOME AT FIRST."

Dentist (*exultantly*). "NOT A BIT OF IT, SIR! LOOK HERE, SIR!" (*Dexterously catching his entire set.*) "HERE'S MY UPPERS, AND HERE'S MY UNDERS!"

In shooting both sets from his mouth, the dentist is demonstrating a trick possible only with the new springless dentures – also, unwittingly, that to wear anything so loose in the mouth must indeed be irksome. The dentist's dress and the furnishings of his surgery are typically mid-nineteenth century. Drawing by Punch, *1860.*

temporary novels. These descriptions reflect a lack of attention to personal appearance that verged on the inconsiderate.

12

Crowns and Bridges

Efficient porcelain crowns date only from the last quarter of the nineteenth century. The pleasure to be derived from this method of filling unsightly gaps comes out in turn-of-the-century letters from the young President Roosevelt[1] to his parents.

> May 19, 1902
>
> After lunch I went to the dentist, and am now minus my front tooth. He cut it off very neatly and painlessly, took impressions of the root and space, and is having the porcelain tip baked. I hope to have it put in next Friday, and in the meantime I shall avoid all society, as I talk with a lithp and look like a thight.

> May 27, 1902
>
> My tooth is no longer a dream, it is an accomplished fact. It was put in on Friday and is perfect in form, color, lustre, texture, etc. I feel like a new person and have already been proposed to by three girls.

Progress in the making of crowns and bridges was retarded for lack of a grinding machine and of a cement that would stay hard in the mouth. Thus, although by the 1880s almost anyone

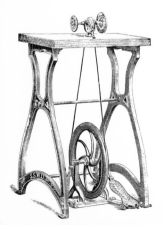

[1] *F.D.R., His Personal Letters*, New York, 1947.

Late nineteenth-century foot-operated dental lathe, much used for grinding porcelain teeth.

could obtain a passable set of full dental plates, even the rich would be fitted with crowns as crude and impermanent as those made in the days of Fauchard. The proper preparation of roots was barely possible with hand instruments. Some dentists were still attaching their crowns with pegs of hickory wood; these were pushed into root canals and held there until the moisture of the mouth caused them to swell and become tight (sometimes roots split). A textbook of 1824 gave these directions:[1]

> A pivot of the toughest wood is inserted, so prepared to enter each cavity without much force, where it will soon swell and make the tooth very permanent and durable. . . . This pivot may be renewed by the patient when necessary.

The first dentist's drill, foot-operated, appeared in 1871; the first satisfactory dental cement (an oxyphosphate of zinc) in 1869. With these two inventions, the one to prepare the parts and the other to stick them together, a range of permanent repairs became possible. Full crowns could now be securely pinned into roots, and jacket crowns, which fit over the filed-down remains of a tooth, at last became a worthwhile restoration. Credit for the first fixed bridge has been given to B.J. Bing of Paris, who fused a gold bar to the back of porcelain teeth – sometimes as many as five in a row.

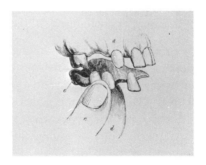

How to place a partial set in the mouth.
From a handbook of 1851.

Most people preferred the fixed replacements because, unlike partial dentures (which usually slipped), they did not carry the full stigma of false teeth. Dentists preferred them, too: they were

[1] Eleazer Gidney, *Treatise on the Teeth.*

more profitable and had the extra advantage that with the new cement they would stay in place even when poorly made. Consequently all roots were saved to hold a bridge. What rarely took place in the nineteenth century was anything in the way of aseptic filling of these roots.

Trouble all too often followed, especially in America where the main mechanical improvements originated. Dr Bremner has written of it as follows in his *Story of Dentistry*:

> Frequently the teeth under the well-constructed bridges would abscess and develop pus-discharging fistulae, but few dentists were disturbed by these manifestations. When a patient expressed some apprehension about tenderness over the root ends, or the flow of some exudate from the gums, he was usually told not to worry about it. The fact that teeth were intimately connected with the blood stream and the nervous system seemed to have escaped the attention not only of the dentist but of the physician as well.

The showdown came in the year 1911. Dr Bremner describes how it arose in a chapter headed 'An Englishman Attacks "American Dentistry" ':

> American dentistry had spread far and wide and was recognized everywhere as the standard of excellence, when suddenly and without any warning, the blow fell. An English physician, William Hunter, publicly accused 'American Dentistry' of contributing to the ill health of the people.

Dr Hunter, practising among the rich of London, had several patients in bed with ailments he was at a loss to diagnose. Some of them, he noticed, had in their mouths extensive restoration work – known as American dentistry – which was dirty and showed supporting roots that appeared unhealthy.

With the idea of giving anything a try, he suggested the removal of the bridges and of the roots holding them. Most of the patients objected. The work had been expensive; removing it meant disfigurement and an impaired chewing mechanism. But of the few who agreed, a significant number began to get rapidly better. Hunter was as surprised as they were. He recorded his observations, and in a paper delivered in Montreal

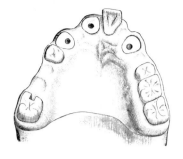
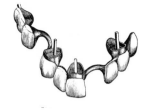

LEFT: *The mouth prepared.*
RIGHT: *The bridge to fit it.*

Late nineteenth-century bridgework of high standard.

to a group of doctors he roundly criticized American dentistry, describing the ingeniously made bridges as 'mausoleums of gold over a mass of sepsis', a phrase to which the Press gave much publicity.

Dentists were indignant, but no arguments could refute the facts underlying Dr Hunter's criticisms. The medical profession became seriously interested; there was fresh thought about the association that exists between the teeth, the gums and the blood stream. Doctors began to believe that although a tooth abscess might do little damage to the face, it could send infectious organisms into the body to lodge in some vital organ or tissue.

Overnight, as it were, they started to blame the teeth for almost any illness they could not readily diagnose. No matter what the patient's trouble, headache or stomach ache, teeth had to come out.

Bewildered dentists took the same line – and were faced with a problem once the teeth had been pulled. It was their job to replace them with false ones, but if bridges and crowns led to bad health, how should they meet patients' demands to have gaps filled? Unlike full dentures, partial ones were inclined to be so loose and uncomfortable that most people refused to wear them.

The bewilderment increased when it was found that wholesale extractions did not always bring recovery. Young people as well as old were having their teeth out, their mouths wrecked and their faces disfigured, without any apparent improvement in their health. Often the psychological effect of losing teeth made them worse.

The increasingly widespread use of X-ray equipment at last brought sanity to the situation. The film showed whether a dead tooth with a filled root was healthy or diseased. Intelligent dentists no longer removed dead teeth which were healthy: they realized that a properly treated tooth without a pulp does not lose its contact with the blood circulation, that it remains a satisfactory part of the anatomy.

13

Transplanting

The barbarous operation of transplanting offered another means of replacing front teeth. Immediately a decayed tooth was drawn a sound one taken from another mouth would be pushed into the vacant socket.

The transplanting of human teeth was referred to by Paré in 1564 and by Charles Allen, with distaste, in 1685. In the late eighteenth century, publicity turned it into a craze. Some dentists did as many as six transplants in a week, though with varying success. The better ones – since disease was occasionally transferred – made some attempt to check that those who offered their teeth were free from infection; and it was thought wise to rinse the newly extracted good tooth in warm water. Under the best circumstances, a transplant would settle down in a month or two and remain firm for three, even five years.

Although a few voices were raised at the cruelty of depriving the poor of useful teeth, no one was surprised that poverty should impel them to earn a little money in this way. There seems never to have been a serious lack of volunteers. Laetitia-Matilda Hawkins writes in her *Memoirs* (1824) that the celebrated Lady Hamilton once resolved to sell some of her front teeth: she was then young Emma Hart, out of a situation and destitute. On her way to the dentist, however, she met an old fellow servant who persuaded her to resort to a less creditable method of making money. In Victor Hugo's *Les Misérables* (1862), Fantine's heart-rending situation obliges her to sell first her hair, then her incisors and finally her virtue.

The writings of John Hunter were largely responsible for the increased popularity of transplanting. His stature as a general surgeon was such that people paid attention to what he said about dentistry. Hunter undertook personally numerous transplantings, a task which he considered, unlike supervision of false-teeth making, within the province of a surgeon.

In his *Natural History of the Human Teeth* he advised operators to have several people in attendance. If the first person's tooth

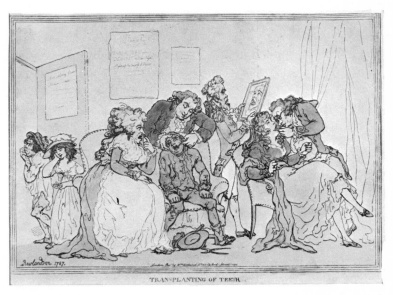

Rowlandson's Transplanting of Teeth *(1787)*. *The chimney sweep's tooth is to be tried for size in the jaw of the fashionable woman sitting beside him on the sofa.*

did not suit, the corresponding one from the next should be instantly pulled and tried in. Once a reasonable fit had been achieved, the transplanted tooth had to be immobilized by tying it to the adjacent ones.

The etching by Thomas Rowlandson (1787) gives an idea of the preposterous procedure. The dentist[1] is shown extracting a tooth from a young chimney sweep sitting beside a fashionably dressed lady whose jaw is about to receive the tooth. She awaits it with smelling salts held to her nose. On the right the next

[1] A caricature of Bartholomew Ruspini.

patient, a girl, sits with clenched hands while an assistant examines her mouth. Behind her, a patient who has been treated regards the result without enthusiasm in a glass. At the far left, two raggedly-dressed young people, holding their aching jaws, are leaving the room. The little girl looks down at the coins taken in payment for her teeth. On the door a sign reads: 'Most money given for "live" teeth'. Another, inside the room, describes the dentist as dentist to the Empress of Russia.

There is something especially pathetic in the way the very young were exploited. But Hunter strongly recommended the teeth of young healthy subjects as those most likely to transplant well. He admitted that by no means every case succeeded. What he meant by success is probably exemplified by the following case history of an American patient of his which has been written up by Dr Menzies Campbell in *The Dental Practitioner*.

Three lower front teeth, he relates, were skilfully transplanted and in a short time became quite firm. Five years later they had worked loose. The man consulted the Philadelphian dentist James Gardette, who found that the upper teeth were biting on them too heavily and causing inflammation. He filed down the transplanted teeth and prescribed an astringent mouthwash. Within two months they were tight again, remained so for a further five years, and subsequently stayed in place for several years in a loose condition.

The transplanting boom spread from Europe to America in the latter years of the eighteenth century. A French surgeon called Pierre Le Mayeur had a lot to do with this by electing to specialize in the operation. He arrived in America in 1781, having spent some years in London, and within five years was prosperous enough to establish a stable of horses. Little would have been known of this plainly genial and interesting man but for meticulous research by Dr Weinberger, the fruits of which appear in his *History of Dentistry in America* (1948).

Le Mayeur treated George Washington several times, staying overnight at Mount Vernon for the purpose. Although there is no record of his having transplanted teeth for Washington, it is known that he transplanted four front teeth and one eye tooth for his aide, Colonel Richard Varick. Washington remarked in a letter to Varick: 'I have been staggered in my belief in the efficacy of transplantation of living teeth.'

For several years from 1782 Le Mayeur regularly advertised in the papers:

> Doctor LE MAYEUR. FRONT TEETH. Any person disposed to part with their FRONT TEETH may receive Two guineas for each Tooth, on applying to No. 28, Maiden Lane [New York].

The price varied between one and five guineas according to the supply. It seems to have been reluctant in Richmond, Virginia, where he made a professional stay. The price there was the top five guineas a tooth, 'slaves' teeth excepted'.

But Le Mayeur did not always take advantage of the offers. There is the evidence of the following anecdote in the *Daily Advertiser* for 28 January 1789, in which he is the dentist referred to:

> In the severe winter of 1783, which was a time of general distress in New York, an aged couple found themselves reduced to their last stick of wood. They were supported by a daughter, who found herself unable to secure wood, fuel or provision. She accidentally heard of a dentist who advertised that he would give 3 guineas for every sound tooth. She decided to do this. On her arrival she made known the circumstances which caused her to make the sacrifice. He, affected by her tears, refused, and presented her with 10 guineas instead.

In the *New York Independent Journal* of 18 December 1784 he announced:

> Dr. Le Mayeur has transplanted one hundred and twenty three teeth since last June, and assures the public that not one of his operations has failed of the wished-for success.

The latter assertion need not be the blatant lie it appears at first sight. As Le Mayeur was writing within a few months of the operations, it is quite possible that in the interval none of the transplanted teeth had gone wrong to the point of having to come out – or if some had, that he had not yet heard about it. And the phrase 'wished-for success' is ingenious: Le Mayeur would have been aware that with certain transplantings a brief life was all the success that he, at any rate, could wish for.

Viewed in this way, Le Mayeur's claim can even be reconciled with a report of 1824, some twenty years after his death, written by his colleague Gardette. Le Mayeur had apparently told Gardette that during a stay in Philadelphia for the winter of 1785–6 he transplanted 170 teeth: 'of these transplanted teeth', states Gardette, 'not one succeeded'. He adds, though, that a few lasted for a year or so. Here is part of the report:

> In the course of my practice, after that time, I had occasion to extract at least fifty of these transplanted teeth – most of them without an instrument, with my fingers only – and to replace them by artificial teeth [He claimed that one such replacement, a human Crown mounted on gold, 'resembled so perfectly the large incisor which remained, that no person could perceive the difference'.] Many accidents occurred to the transplanted teeth, while they were growing firm, and some never got firmly fixed in the sockets at all.

However, Gardette was writing to a thesis: he called his paper *Observations on the Transplantation of Teeth, which tend to show the Impossibility of the Success of that Operation*. His argument is that transplanting could only work, as replacing a tooth in its

W A N T E D.

FRONT TEETH, for which Two Guineas a piece will be given, by J. BROWNE, Surgeon and Dentist, No. 6, Naſſau-Street.
New-York, Sept. 29, 1784.   87

Advertisement in the New York City Directory, *1786.*

own socket worked (replantation), if the root of the transplant was exactly the length, size and shape of the defective one; and as this was a matter the dentist had to decide without seeing either, it was impossible.

In England, Berdmore and William Rae, both dentists of

distinction and appointed to serve George III, had expressed themselves opponents of transplanting. Berdmore called the operation 'dangerous and immoderately expensive' and considered, anyway, that the apparently successful transplantings were really replantings: the operator had quickly filled and repaired the extracted bad tooth and then put it back again, charging the fee for a transplanted tooth. Berdmore said he had seen the evidence of this deception in the mouths of his patients. In Rae's opinion, a tooth cruelly drawn from an impoverished person was especially liable to disease.

It would be seemly to report that transplanting quickly died out as the nineteenth century wore on and as false teeth improved. But although the craze was over, some rich people, especially women, continued to insist on the operation. As late as 1919 in *Dental Surgery and Pathology* J.F. Colyer sets out the method of performing it. The patient to receive the transplanted tooth

> is first operated upon, as little injury as possible being inflicted, and the bleeding from the socket arrested as far as possible. The tooth to be transplanted is next removed from the other patient and immediately transferred to the vacant socket and forced well into place. Union in transplantation may be a process similar to that which takes place in replantation, or the process may be entirely different . . . absorption of portions of the root taking place first.

However, Colyer, who was examiner in dentistry to the Royal College of Surgeons, does put forward the moral objection that 'the teeth to be transplanted are usually obtained from the poorer classes', and opines that, considering everything, the practice is to be condemned. Since Colyer's day the only sort of transplanting that has been publicly discussed is the more respectable procedure of shifting teeth about within the same mouth. Replanting teeth dislodged by accident remains accepted practice; it almost always succeeds if resorted to without delay.

14

False Teeth for the Masses

Of the multitudes who never dreamed of buying false teeth, many got on well enough once all their own teeth and projecting stumps had finally departed. Thomas Hardy wrote in Chapter fifteen of *Far From the Madding Crowd* that

> The maltster's lack of teeth appeared not to sensibly diminish his powers as a mill. He had been without them for so many years that toothlessness was felt less to be a defect than hard gums an acquisition.

But though adequate mastication could be achieved, over-closing of the lower jaw sometimes brought on deafness.

The era of false teeth for the masses began in the 1850s with the American invention of sulphur-hardened rubber – that is, vulcanite – for moulding the bases. Accurate wax impressions of a toothless mouth had been possible since the beginning of the nineteenth century, and gold (which does not stain) was sometimes beaten out on metal casts to make plates that were much better than those of carved ivory; but the process, especially the fixing of the individual artificial teeth, was lengthy,

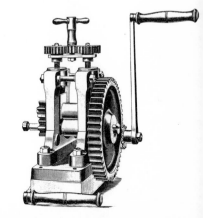

Nineteenth-century hand mill for rolling gold ingots into sheets for dental plates.

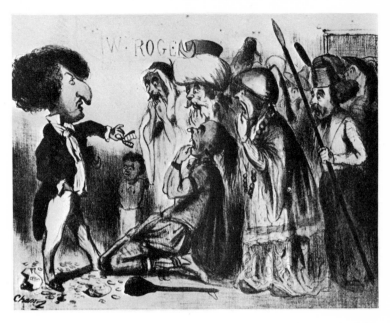

Caricature by C. H. Amadée de Noé. William Rogers, dentist, demonstrating false teeth in the East. c. 1855.

intricate and very expensive. Charles Goodyear's vulcanite, on the other hand, was cheap and easy to work.

The new material was given an excellent start by appearing only a few years after the introduction of anaesthesia, which had caused an unprecedented demand for false teeth. Numerous people who had preferred toothache to the torture of extraction were now hastening to have rotten teeth cleared from their mouths. The American dentist Dr Bremner graphically describes the situation in his *Story of Dentistry* and observes:

> If the entire profession had devoted its efforts exclusively to the making of false teeth, it could not have supplied the demand with the means and methods available. . . . It is hard to imagine what the profession would have done had not Goodyear discovered the vulcanization process.

Anaesthesia by inhaling was discovered by Horace Wells, a young dentist of Hartford, Connecticut. In December 1844, he attended a public entertainment on the amusing effects of laughing gas (nitrous oxide) at which volunteer inhalers would laugh or sing or fight according to their temperaments. The local newspaper's advertisement assured its readers:

> Eight Strong Men are engaged to occupy the front seats to protect those under the influence of the Gas, from injuring themselves or others. . . . No language can described the delightful sensation produced. . . . N.B. The gas will only be administered to gentlemen of the first respectability. The object is to make the entertainment a genteel affair.

A friend of Wells who climbed on the platform became so pugnacious that even eight strong men could not prevent him from crashing violently into the back of a bench. The shock sobered him and he stumbled back to his seat beside Wells, not noticing that blood was pouring from what turned out to be a wide gash in his leg. He said he had felt nothing.

Looking at the wound, Wells became suddenly excited. Surely this gas could be used for the painless extraction of teeth? That very evening he went round to discuss the idea with a dentist friend called Riggs, also of Hartford. Riggs has left an account of what ensued:

> Wells and I had a conference that night and determined to try the gas on Wells the next morning. . . . Wells took his seat in the operating chair. I examined the tooth so as to be ready to operate without delay. Wells took the bag in his lap – held the tube to his mouth and inhaled till insensibility relaxed the muscles of his arms – his hands fell on his breast – his head dropped on the headrest, and I instantly passed the forceps into the mouth – onto the tooth and extracted it.

Four witnesses were standing in the doorway

> ready to run out if Wells jumped up from the chair and made any hostile demonstrations. You may ask why he did not get up? Simply because he could not. Our agreement, the night previous, was to push the administration to a point hitherto unknown. We knew not whether death or success confronted us. It was *terra incognita* we were bound to explore; the result is known to the world. No one but Wells and myself knew to what point the inhalation was to be carried – the result was painfully

problematical to us but the great law of Nature, hitherto unknown, was kind to us, and a grand discovery was born into the world.

On coming to, Wells is reported to have said: 'I did not feel it so much as the prick of a pin. That was the first tooth drawn without pain.' He straightway began to use the gas in his practice. On 20 January 1845, a Boston newspaper printed the following item:

> A dentist in Hartford, Connecticut, has adopted the use of nitrous oxide gas in tooth pulling. It is said that after taking this gas the patient feels no pain.

Friends urged Wells to patent the discovery, but he said, 'No, let it be free as the air.' He was an emotional and expansive young man and sadly did not live to see the extent of the benefit he had conferred on humanity. He took to doing himself for fun with another gas, chloroform, and became an addict. One day 'coming out of a stupor and exhilarated beyond measure', as he wrote in a letter, he seized a phial of acid from the mantel, rushed into the street and threw its contents at two prostitutes plying their trade there. He was arrested but managed to commit suicide, writing in his final note: 'Oh, my dear mother, brother and sister, what can I say to you? My anguish will only allow me to bid farewell.' Wells died, leaving a wife and child, three years after making his wonderful discovery.

Before long people were flocking to have teeth pulled out on hearing that a whiff or two of gas made the operation painless. The employment of vulcanite in fitting them out with replacements swept the United States.

But, unlike anaesthesia, it was by no means as free as air. The Goodyear Rubber Company had several patents assigned to it and was determined to make a fortune out of dentists using its process. Fees ranged from 25 to 100 dollars a year, depending on the size of the practice, plus a royalty of two dollars for each denture containing six or more teeth. There was widespread annoyance. Thousands of dentists accepted the terms, but plenty tried to conceal their use of vulcanite.

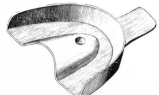

Tray for conveying impression material into the mouth. Nineteenth century.

These were sought out by agents of the company who travelled widely and did all they could to enforce the patent claims by intimidation and lawsuits. A notice in the Jacksonville, Illinois *Journal* illustrates the methods employed; it was inserted by one Josiah Bacon, described as treasurer of the Hard Rubber Company of Boston:

> Drs. Widenham and Cary are duly authorized licencees in Morgan County for using vulcanite bases for mounting artificial teeth. We warn all dentists infringing on our patent and all persons employing them that they will be prosecuted to the full extent of the law.

The company had amassed over three million dollars when, on 13 April 1879, Bacon was murdered in a San Francisco hotel bedroom by an irate dentist who had twice been in trouble for infringement. As a result, pugnacious methods of collection ceased. Two years later the patents expired, leaving dentists at last free to make any use of rubber that they pleased.

Vulcanite was not in fact an ideal material for dental plates. Slightly porous, it was hard to clean, held the taste of certain

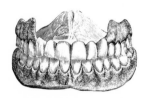 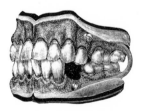

LEFT: *Late nineteenth-century full set – vulcanite.*
RIGHT: *Late nineteenth-century full set with springs and a rubber attachment.*

foods and sometimes caused soreness. The colour of the gumwork was so flat and unnatural that it became usual when this part showed – and when the patient could afford it – to attach porcelain gum to the front of the bases. For this purpose dental manufacturers supplied sections of two or three false teeth with the gum as part of them. They were not always used with discrimination, and in *Mechanical Dentistry* (1897 edition), the American dentist Joseph Richardson writes:

The indiscriminate and almost universal employment of block or sectional gum teeth in connection with rubber has done more to degrade the prosthetic department of dental practice than all other causes combined. The optional arrangement of each individual tooth to meet the requirements of special cases is one of the absolute and indispensable requirements of a perfect artificial denture.

One good result of the vulcanite patent business was that dentists were encouraged to try out new materials for cheap bases (gold stayed the best of the expensive ones[1]), and thus avoid the annoying payments. Celluloid was hailed with enthusiasm by some dentists. It was brittle and had a tendency to warp and to turn gradually from pink to green; but as the years went by improved forms of the material did make it eventually an acceptable alternative to vulcanite.

Celluloid is of course inflammable, hardly a major disadvantage, but one that is thought to have been the undoing of Sir Compton Mackenzie's friend, mentioned in Chapter 1, whose false teeth caught on fire when he fell asleep with the end of a lighted cigarette between his lips.

Vulcanite continued in use far into the twentieth century and long after celluloid and various metals had been found wanting. It was recently superseded by the acrylic resins which are commonly used for both plates and teeth. These plastic teeth are made to look extremely pleasant, at last realizing the eighteenth-century boast, 'not to be distinguish'd from natural', and have the single disadvantage of being rather soft. Some say, however, that the gradual abrasion is a good point, since it enables each person to wear down his teeth into the relationship best suited to his own jaw movements.

---

[1] Gold plates were pawnable (for their intrinsic value). Dame Edith Sitwell, whose mother had financial difficulties, used to talk of being sent out at the age of seventeen to pawn parental false teeth. The story appears in John Lehmann's *A Nest of Tigers*, 1968.

15

False Teeth in
Eighteenth-century America

Little restorative dentistry went on in eighteenth-century colonial America, despite the immigration towards the end of the century of various dentists from England and the Continent. Even Martha Washington, wife of the President, seemed unable to get prompt attention. Correspondence assembled by Dr Weinberger shows her at one period with broken-down false teeth, waiting in vain for new ones to arrive.[1]

Some time in 1797 Mrs Washington ordered a row of teeth from Benjamin Fendall, whose lecture-like advertisements she may have seen in the papers. Dr Fendall, as he called himself, was a prolific writer of advertisements, the main material for which was lifted straight from Berdmore's *Disorders and Deformities of the Teeth*. Fendall's 'case wherein he extirpated an excrescence, in the mouth of a young lady, as large as an Indian Walnut' is word for word from Berdmore except for the substitution of young lady for young man.

Mrs Washington's teeth were late in arriving, and on 6 March 1798, the President himself wrote to him:

Sir
    Mrs Washington has been long in expectation of receiving what you took away unfinished, and was to have completed and sent to her: – and prays that it may be done without further delay, as she is in want of them and must apply elsewhere, if not done.

The following letter was received from Fendall a year and five months later:

[1] B.H. Weinberger, *History of Dentistry in America*, St Louis, 1948.

Dr. Sir

Within this Day, or two, I found myself, so much relieved, from my long continued and painful illness, tho I use my left arm, with some difficulty, as to be enabled to finish Mrs. Washingtons Teeth, and you'll receive them, safe, I hope, by my Servant, They are as nearly as I can now, recollect – like the old ones as there are so many ways, to make and shape Teeth – twou'd be almost impossible, to make them, exactly alike – after some time, without having the old ones present. The model, I took, has, also, by accident, sustained some injury. I am extremely sorry, indeed, yr Lady has been obliged to wait so long – owing to my long absence from home and my Illness, after I had arrived at Cedar-Hill. I wish you and Mrs Washington to have every conviction within yourself, I ever will with promptitude, and with pleasure, serve you both, whenever you may choose to command me – if in my power, and I fondly flatter myself, you'll both deem my excuse to be sufficiently admissible – at this Time. Please to present my most respectful comp. to Mrs Washington & believe me, Dr. Sir.

Yrs with due respect,

B. Fendall.

The teeth were enclosed with a request that the General should hand Fendall's servant twenty-eight dollars on delivery.

In the meantime Mrs Washington had written to a dentist in Philadelphia, Charles Whitelock – who was also an actor:

Mrs Washington will be much obliged to Mr Whitelock to make for her a set of teeth – to make her some thing bigger and thicker in the front and a some matter longer.

She will be very glad if he will do them soon, as those she has is almost broak.

But there was no response. Whitelock was in Boston, and busier with acting than with dentistry.

He had arrived from England in 1794 and, like other dentists, moved round from one town to another, announcing his arrival in the local paper. In 1794 he respectfully informed

the Ladies and Gentlemen of Baltimore and its vicinity that he continues to perform all operations on the Teeth – Supplies the deficiencies of nature with Artificial or Real Teeth, in all the various modes of fixing. . . . He waits upon Ladies and Gentlemen at their houses.

According to his list of charges, fixings used were ligatures, gold screws or gold sockets: artificial teeth five dollars each, human ones seven dollars.

The first full set of false teeth fitted in America is attributed to Robert Wooffendale, a Yorkshireman. It was worn by one William Walton of New York and apparently met his highest

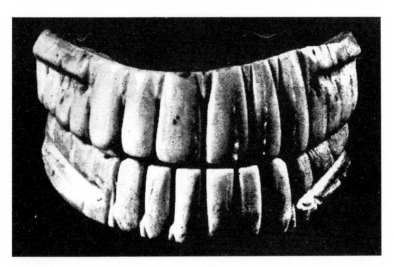

Full set of ivory teeth by Robert Wooffendale. c. 1768. Similar to the set made for William Walton – the first ever fitted in America.

expectations. In the words of a mid nineteenth-century dental journal, it 'was thought to be a wonderful triumph of genius'. Wooffendale's first advertisement ran as follows:

Robert Woffendale [he later changed the spelling], SURGEON DENTIST, lately arrived from London (who was instructed by Thomas Berdmore, Esq; Operator for the Teeth to his present Britanick Majesty), begs leave to inform the Public, that he performs all Operations upon the Teeth, Gums, Sockets, and Palate: Likewise fixes artificial Teeth so as to escape Discernment, and without pain, or the least inconvenience.

N.B. May be spoke with at his Lodgings, at Mr. John Laboyteaux, at the Golden Ball, betwixt the Fly Market and the New Dutch Church (New York), from the Hours of nine in the Morning to six in the Evening.

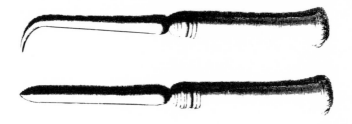

Instruments for removing decay. Eighteenth century.

False teeth were sometimes hard to come by in eighteenth-century America and it was not unknown for sensitive people to try their hand at making at least partial sets for themselves. Charles Willson Peale, the fashionable portrait painter, naturalist, lecturer and founder of the Philadelphia Academy of Fine Arts, made his own full upper and lower dentures. He made a set for his son Rembrandt, when the latter was twenty-eight – and also for various friends.

Rembrandt Peale (d. 1860) wrote as follows for the *New American Encyclopedia:*

> My father, Charles W. Peale, at an early age losing his teeth, supplied himself with artificial ones made of ivory, as usual. But about the year 1807, reading in the newspapers some account of what was then called 'mineral teeth', he employed himself in making many experiments to ascertain the best composition – procuring the finest Chinese clay, silex, and platina filings . . . and finally furnished himself and some of his friends with the first porcelain teeth that were made in America.

Although never acting professionally as a dental mechanic, Peale has been allowed a place in dental histories. Dr Bremner writes in *The Story of Dentistry*: 'Credit for being the first to bake mineral teeth in the U.S.A. probably belongs to Charles W. Peale.'

Peale lived to be eighty-six. In his eightieth year he wrote an autobiography in the third person and says of his home-made false teeth that

> the mode of executing them . . . was first to form a plate of pure silver to fit the gums exactly and then to solder a thin plate round

each plate that fitted the gums in a perpendicular position, on the front of this plate the teeth is riveted – a single rivet was generally sufficient, and to put springs to keep the teeth in their place, he was much indebted to his friend Mr John Dorsey. . . . Mr Dorsey's invention of springs [was] greatly superior to any invention before used, as they permitted the jaws to open to the fullest extent and also every grinding motion. . . .

For the actual teeth, he tried several animal substances before discovering the virtues of porcelain. Ivory, from whatever source, he found very liable to offensive decay, leading to 'great loss of time by a repetition of the work'. This 'made him try to find a harder substance in Horses and Cows teeth, of which he made a great number of teeth but the hardest of teeth he found belonged to Hogs, but they could very seldom be had sufficiently large. . . .'

Advice on do-it-yourself false teeth – or what would serve as such – was published by at least one American dentist, B.T. Longbottom, who writes in *Treatise on Dentistry* (1802) – under the heading 'Artificial Teeth' – that since

many have succeeded in making them, I know no objection to others giving it a trial; the best way to which is, impressing of wax, so as to form and fit the vacated space. At first it will carry an awkward appearance, but by repeated parings, become more shapeable and resembling the thing wanted, and may serve as a model, for yourself to fashion one more substantial. . . .

In 1802 dentistry to the American public at large still meant no more than tooth-drawing and tooth scraping. Longbothom observes in his preface:

Though the subject is in some measure new here, I yet hope for every reasonable indulgence, having received the general approbation of the most eminent professors in surgery and medicine, who have not hesitated to assert its great utility. . . .

16

George Washington

George Washington, first president of the United States, suffered for most of his life from the inadequacies of eighteenth-century dental treatment. There was recurrent toothache, tormenting him during the Revolutionary War; there was the mental suffering of a man acutely sensitive about his appearance.

Washington had the sort of teeth that decay fast and need prompt repair work. This was not to be had. Despite buying sponge tooth-brushes by the dozen, he lost one tooth after another from the age of twenty-two. His soldiering friend George Mercer mentions defective teeth in a description of him at twenty-eight and says he generally kept his mouth firmly closed.[1]

From his early forties, Washington was struggling with partial dentures held in with wire ligatures – for which the necessary equipment was not always to hand. In March 1781 he wrote as follows to John Baker, a dentist of Philadelphia:[2]

A day or two ago I requested Colo. Harrison to apply to you for a pair of Pincers to fasten the wire of my teeth. – I hope you furnished him with them. – I now wish you would send me one of your scrapers, as my teeth stand in need of cleaning, and I have little prospect of being in Philadelphia soon. It would come very safe by Post – and in return, the money shall be sent so soon as I have the cost of it.

Pathetically, this letter never arrived. It was intercepted by

[1] John Hill Morgan, *The Life Portraits of Washington*, 1931.
[2] Letter in the William L. Clements Library, Michigan.

the British – and subsequently held for generations in the family of General Clinton.

Within a few years Washington had lost all but one of his own teeth, a lower pre-molar, and had acquired several false sets made by a variety of so-called dentists. His adopted son,

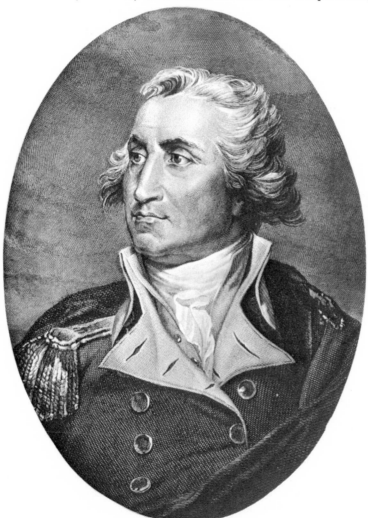

Washington as he looked before wearing full sets of teeth. Portrait by John Trumball.

George Custis, wrote of them 'answering very imperfectly the purpose for which they were intended'.[1] One of the first had bases of lead alloy coated with beeswax; the upper teeth came from some animal, in Dr Weinberger's opinion an elk, while the lower ones were human. The complete set weighs three ounces. Its springs of coiled steel are so powerful that even today several strands of wire are needed to keep the upper and lower parts in contact.

Possibly Washington was wearing this set when he received an English traveller in 1790. The latter wrote:[2]

> His mouth was like no other I ever saw; the lips firm and the under jaw seemed to grasp the upper with force, as if the muscles were in full action when he sat still.

The one remaining tooth at least checked a tendency of lower dentures to move outwards under the thrust of ill-placed springs. But it was loosened in doing this; and from time to time it ached and the surrounding gum swelled up. Washington never cared to remove his teeth, as others did, for the table, and he could not remove the lower set alone since it anchored the springs which supported the top set. He kept these things to himself. When barely recovered from a gruesome bout of gum inflammation, he gave a large dinner. Senator William Maclay, who was present, recorded in his journal:

> The President seemed to bear in his countenance a settled aspect of melancholy. No cheering ray of sunshine broke through the cloudy gloom of settled seriousness. At every interval of eating and drinking he played on the table with a fork or a knife, like a drumstick.

(This was not the first reference to banging on the table with cutlery.)

An English manufacturer called Henry Wansey, who breakfasted at his house a few years later in 1794, wrote of 'a certain anxiety visible in his countenance, with marks of extreme sensibility'.[3] The meal had been sliced tongue and bread and

---

[1] Hill Morgan.   [2] Hill Morgan.
[3] Stephen Dacatur, Jr., *Private Affairs of George Washington*, Boston, 1933.

butter. For private consumption, Washington like pickled tripe. He once wrote personally to the head of a London firm of merchants asking him to ship over a supply. 'Dental infirmity', he explained, 'impels me caring for this necessary item in our domestic commissariat.'

In 1796 it at last became necessary to part with the one remaining natural tooth (it is today in a gold case at the New

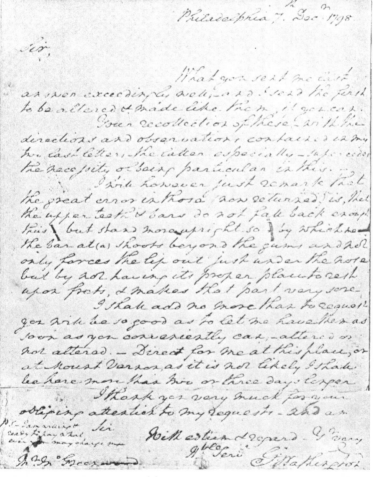

A letter from Washington to Greenwood with instructions about the inclination of the front false teeth.

York Academy of Medicine). As the gum ridge had become flattened, there was now nothing but Washington's face muscles to hold back the lower teeth. To reduce the protrusion, he attacked the front of at least one lower denture with a file. Upper sets also gave extra trouble. Returning one to a dentist for alteration, he complained[1]

> it shoots beyond the gums and not only forces the lip out just under the nose but by not having its proper place to rest upon frets, and makes that part very sore.

Chewing must have become almost impossible. But Washington could put up with discomfort; and he was probably unaware that his dental state contributed to the indigestion and short temper he began to suffer, and that the unnatural motions of the lower jaw were the likely cause of his deafness. What did upset him was the change in the shape of his face and in his articulation; he became reluctant to speak in public. Maclay wrote that artificial teeth made the voice hollow and indistinct.

In letters to John Greenwood, the dentist he now used regularly, he expresses decided views on how the front teeth should be inclined. Here is an example dated Philadelphia, 7 December 1798:[2]

> Sir,
> Your letter of 8th came safe – and as I am hurrying in order to leave this city tomorrow, I must be short.
> The principal thing you will have to attend to, in the alteration you will have to make, is to let the upper bar fall back from the lower one thus *; whether the teeth are quite straight, or inclining a little in thus * or a little rounding outward thus * is immaterial, for I find it is the bars alone, both above and below, that gives the lips the pointing and swelling appearance – of consequence, if this can be remedied, all will be well.
> I send the old bars, which you have returned to me with the new set, because you have desired. – But they may be destroyed, or anything else done with them you please, for you will find that I have been obliged to file them away so much above, to remedy

---

[1] Letter in the Library of Congress.
[2] Letter in the Old South Meeting House, Boston.

the evil I have been complaining of as to render them useless perhaps to receive new teeth. – But of this you are better able to judge than I am. – If you can fix the teeth (new on the new bars which you have) on the old bars which you will receive with this letter I should prefer it because the latter are easy in the mouth, and you will perceive moreover that when the edge of the upper and lower teeth are put together that the upper falls back into the mouth, which they ought to do, or it will have the effect of forcing the lip out just under the nose.

I shall only repeat again, that I feel much obliged by your extreme willingness, and readiness to accommodate me, and that I am, Sir,

Your Obedt Servant
Go. Washington

The teeth sent back are those shown in the illustration. The lower set's base had been so worn away by filing that it had become flat underneath instead of having a U-shape to fit over the gums. One side of the denture being longer than the other was the result of modification later when Washington's last remaining tooth, loosened by the appliance, had to be pulled out.

Replaceable ivory teeth in two solid sections are attached to

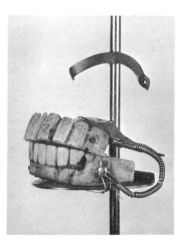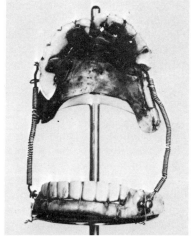

LEFT: *Teeth worn by George Washington – now in the care of Baltimore Dental College.*
RIGHT: *Another view of the teeth (Baltimore).*

this base with wooden dowels that pierce it. The upper teeth, also represented by two sections of ivory, are mounted with plates and rivets to a plate of swaged gold – a form of upper base new at the time.

Greenwood wrote to Washington from New York on 28 December 1798:[1]

Sir,

I send you inclosed two setts of teeth, one fixed on the Old Barrs in part and the sett you sent me from philadelphia which when I Received was very black. Ocationed either by your soaking them in port wine, or by your drinking it.[2] Port wine being sower takes of all the polish, and All Acids has a tendency to soften every kind of teeth and bone. Acid is used in Couloring every kind of Ivory, therefore it is very pernicious to the teeth. I Advice you to either take them out After dinner and put them in clean water and put in another sett, or clean them with a brush and som chalk scraped fine. it will Absorb the Acids which Collects from the mouth and preserve them longer – I have found another and better way of using the sealing wax when holes is eaten in the teeth by acids & – first observe and dry the teeth, then take a piece of Wax and Cut it into as small pieces as you think will fill up the hole, then, take a large nail or any other piece of Iron and heat it hot into the fier. then put your piece of wax into the hole and melt it by means of introduceing the point of the Nail to it. I have tried it and found it to Consoladate and do better than the other way and if done proper it will resist the Saliva. it will be handyer for you to take hold of the Nail with small plyers than with a tongs. Thus the wax must be very small not bigger than this *, if your teeth Grows black, take some chalk and a Pine or Cedar stick, it will rub it of. If you whant your teeth more yellower soak them in Broath or pot liquer, but not in tea or Acids. Porter is a Good thing to Coulor them and will not hurt but preserve them but it must not be in the least pricked – You will find I have Altered the upper teeth you sent me from philadelphia leaveing the enamel on the teeth dont preserve them any longer then if it was of, it only holds the colour better. but to preserve them they must be very often Changed and Cleaned for whatever atacks them must be repelled as Often, or it will gain

---

[1] Letter in the keeping of the Pennsylvania Historical Society.

[2] According to the American dental historian Karl C. Wold, Washington soused his teeth in port to check their disagreeable taste.

ground and destroy the works – the two setts I repaired is done on a different plan than when they are done when made entirely new, for the teeth are forward on the barrs, instead of having the barrs cast red hot on them, which is the reason I believe the destroy or desolve so soone, near to the barrs.

Sir, After hoping you will not be Obliged to be troubled very sune in the same Way. I Subscribe myselvth Your very humble servant,

John Greenwood

Sir, The Additional Charge is fiveteen dollars. P.S. I Expect next spring to move my family into Connecticut State. if I do. I will rite. and let you know. . . . I will as long as I live do any thing in this way for you or in any other way in my power if you require it.

Washington thought highly of Greenwood, and acknowledged receipt of this letter and of the false teeth in terms which

J. GREENWOOD,

DENTIST TO THE LATE PRESIDENT

GEORGE WASHINGTON,

Informs the Public, that he continues to perform every operation incident to the TEETH and GUMS, from the fixing-in of a single tooth to a complete set. The approbation which the late ILLUSTRIOUS WASHINGTON was pleased to bellow on him, he flatters himself, is a sufficient recommendation of his abilities as a Dentist.

Extract from General Washington's Letter.

" January 6, 1799.
" I shall always prefer your services to that of any other in the line of your present profession."

N. B. His prices are very moderate, as no person can exceed him in facility and neatness of performance.

☞ J. GREENWOOD may be consulted at his house, No. 13 PARK, which is the fourth door (towards St. Paul's Church) from the Theatre.

Advertisement by John Greenwood in the New York City Directory, 1800 – less than a year after Washington's death.

105

Greenwood was able to make use of, later on, in his advertisements:[1]

> I feel obliged to you for your attention to my request and for the directions you have given me.
>
> Enclosed you will find bank notes for fifteen dollars, which I should be glad to hear have got safe to your hands. If you should remove to Connecticut, I should be glad to be advised of it, and to what place, as I shall always prefer your services to those of any other in the line of your present profession.

The effect of uncouth false teeth on Washington's appearance is still to be seen all over the world in the picture of his face on American paper money and stamps. Gilbert Stuart, who did

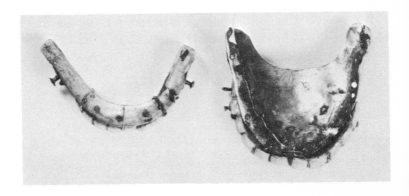

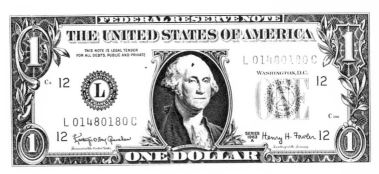

ABOVE: *Washington's teeth again. Note foreshortening of lower bar.*
BELOW: *how his image is most often seen today.*

[1] Weinberger.

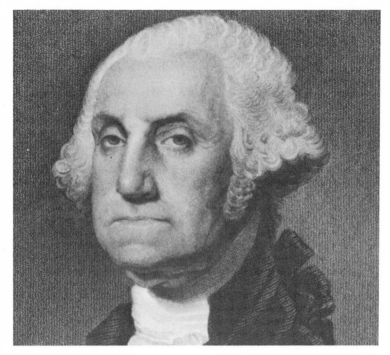

Washington wearing Greenwood's teeth. Portrait by Gilbert Stuart, 1796.

the original portrait, tried to soften the protrusion of the lower teeth by getting Washington to put rolls of cotton in his mouth: the result was the addition of a curious plumpness towards the chin where there should have been a concave curve. Some think it a pity that more use has not been made of a portrait done before all the natural teeth were lost, the one reproduced on the 1922 quarter-dollar piece.

Dentistry has been important in the lives of other United States presidents. President Grover Cleveland (d. 1908) had to have one entire upper jaw removed in addition to most of his teeth – the operation was done aboard his yacht to keep it secret from the nation – and was furnished with an appliance which allowed him to talk and eat with the best. His appearance was positively improved.[1]

[1] Robert Hilkene, in *Bulletin of the History of Dentistry*, Chicago, 1965.

The plate and artificial jaw of vulcanized rubber seemed to Grover Cleveland miraculous. When his dentist, Kasson Gibson of New York, sent along a replacement for the initial temporary appliance, he wrote in acknowledgement:

> I hasten to announce that you have scored another dental victory. The new plate came last night – I looked at it askance. I put it in this morning and I have worn it all day with the utmost ease and comfort and without a shred of packing. I took it out to cleanse it after breakfast and lunch, but found very little on or behind it that needed attention.

President Jackson (d. 1845) had two full sets of teeth made for him but, finding them objectionable, declined ever to wear them. He spoke in public as little as possible and appears frankly toothless in the portraits.[1]

[1] Hilkene.

17

Nineteenth-century Tricks of the Trade

Dentists in general had a bad name throughout the nineteenth century – and not only because of the pain they had to inflict. It was all too easy for the least trained person to put a sign above his door and for toothache or unsightly gaps to drive the unsuspecting inside; tyros and impostors advertised alongside the reputable dentists, exactly copying their phrases.

Proper training, it must in fairness be said, was hard to come by; until 1858 no dental school existed in England. A young man had to be apprenticed to an established dentist for a premium of around £300 to £500 for a five-year indenture; his master, jealous of his methods and working in isolation, would bind him (as of course other craftsmen bound their apprentices) not to divulge secrets of the practice.

The reputable and honest dentists campaigned endlessly against the charlatans; it was a losing battle. John Gray, a member of the Royal College of Surgeons, wrote in 1838 of

the great number of adventurers who have lately assumed the character of dentists without being either surgeons or mechanics. . . . The greatest mischiefs inflicted by quacks is the odium and distrust their malpractices bring upon the profession they invade. Scarcely a week passes in which I am not consulted by some person who has been entrapped . . . and made to pay for an injury: and as the fear of exposure on the part of the sufferer precludes all application for redress, the impostor continues his career in security.

In the same year, in the magazine *Town*, it was observed that[1]

[1] Menzies Campbell.

dentistry, as we find it called, is growing into a profession which numbers nearly as many members as surgery. Great rogues many of them are.

There is a record[1] of a gentleman of Colchester being beguiled by advertisements of high skill and low charges to patronize a travelling dental expert who had arrived in the town – in fact a charlatan whose legitimate occupation was baking. He simply wished, he told him, to have two holes filled and one tooth drawn.

The dental expert observed that it was fortunate he had not delayed in consulting him, because in another week it would have been too late to fill the two teeth. While he mixed what he called his patent cement (silver filings and mercury), he spoke of his wide clientele, which seemed to- include most of the nobility.

Having rapidly poured in the filling material, he seated his patient on the floor and gripped the head between his knees. The tooth came out only after a prolonged wrestle and was accidentally accompanied by the tooth next to it. The dental expert said this was fortunate as both teeth were 'ossified'; he hoped the operation had not hurt much. The patient gasped out that he had been nearly murdered, but did hand over the six guineas now asked for.

The situation was not remedied by the passing of the Dentists Act of 1878. This established a Register of existing practitioners and laid it down that in future no one without dental or medical qualifications could be registered, or use the title 'dentist' or 'dental practitioner'. The weakness of the Act was its failure to make it unlawful for the unregistered to practise; all they had to do was to avoid the forbidden titles.

Thus the majority of men offering dental treatment were still more or less charlatans and often illiterate. Indeed, their number increased year by year. They successfully deluded the public by calling themselves 'dental specialists' and 'dental consultants' or 'dental experts'; they put up enormous signs reading Dental Parlour, Dental Surgery or Artificial Teeth;

---

[1] Menzies Campbell.

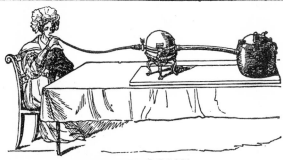

TOOTH-ACHE.

MR. LOCK continues to CURE the TOOTH-ACHE by fumigation or steam from foreign herbs, which has the effect of destroying the nerve without causing any pain to the patient. The cure is effected in three seconds, the tooth remains firm in the socket, and will not decay any further. The patient will, after this operation, be able to draw into the mouth the external air, strike the teeth together, or hold cold water in the mouth, without any pain. The advertiser has a tooth cured 15 years, therefore he can warrant the cure this length of time.—362, Oxford-street, three doors below the Pantheon. Letters post paid. Reference given if required. Charges moderate, according to the circumstances of the patients. This method is not injurious to the health or teeth.

some augmented their newspaper advertisements with posters at railway stations and handbills pushed into the windows of rich people's carriages and under the front doors of big houses.

A mountebank who penetrated the back door of such a house, in person, later sued a maidservant for services rendered. It came out in evidence that he had approached her in a pantry, inspected her teeth, and announced that several needed attention. He then proceeded without permission to break them off at the gums. Profuse bleeding did not deter him from taking a beeswax impression of the mouth with a view to supplying false teeth – for which he frightened the girl into consenting to pay £3 15s. It was stated that she afterwards suffered excruciating pain. Her only consolation was to hear the action dismissed and the man severely reprimanded.[1]

Unregistered persons were prohibited, according to the Act, from recovering in the courts any fee 'for the performance of any dental operation or for any dental attendance or advice,' but it was found that the prohibition could not be made to apply to charges for false teeth.

[1] Menzies Campbell.

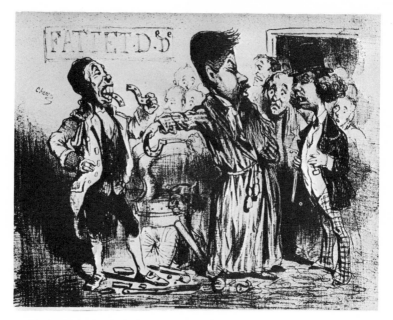

Caricature by C. H. de Amadée de Noé. George Fattett, dentist, hands his servant iron pieces to break with Fattett teeth. c. 1855.

For every kind of operator the main profits came from false teeth; the unqualified man entirely relied on them. Scant knowledge of how to make them need not deter him, for having taken an impression of the mouth he would employ a practised carver to do the rest. Later in the century, with the coming of vulcanite, there grew up several firms of dental mechanics all competing for orders to turn out dental plates to match mouth impressions received. In those days the accepted use of retention springs and ligatures made a perfect fit inessential.

Although taking trouble to decorate their windows with specimen sets of false teeth, most operators, qualified, un-qualified and impostors, worked in humble alleys and courts. This may have been partly to spare the blushes of patients anxious not to be observed making their visits; it did nothing to raise the mean status of dentistry.

Some of the more pushing and ambitious of the London

dentists on the other hand (again, dental 'experts' as well as registered practitioners), paid handsomely to rent rooms at addresses smart enough for anyone to enter with dignity. Such rooms were attended by footmen in livery and contained Turkey carpets, rosewood furniture, magnificent candelabra and expensive paintings and books.

In these surroundings the rich were prepared to pay the frockcoated dentist enormous sums for his false teeth. Dr Menzies Campbell, whose collection of old dental anecdotes is

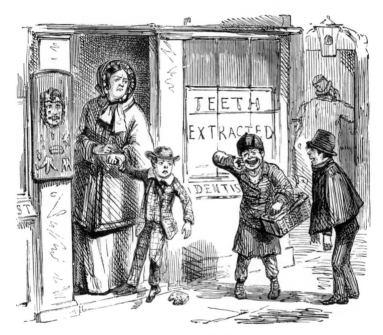

EVIL COMMUNICATIONS.

(AFTER A GREAT DEAL OF COAXING AND PERSUASION, MASTER TOM IS PREVAILED UPON TO PAY HIS QUARTERLY VISIT TO THE DENTIST. INCONSIDERATE AND VULGAR STREET BOYS UNFORTUNATELY PASS AT THE MOMENT HIS OBJECTIONS ARE OVERCOME.)

First Inconsiderate Street Boy. "OH CRIKEY! IF HERE AIN'T A CHAP GOIN' TO HAVE A GRINDER OUT. MY EYE, WHAT FANGS!"

Second Inconsiderate Do. Do. "OH, I WOULDN'T BE 'IM. WON'T THERE BE A SCR-E-W-A-U-N-CH NEETHER!"

[And of course MASTER TOM relapses into his previous very obstinate state.

Typical nineteenth-century dental surgery, looking like a shop. Punch, c. *1880.*

unrivalled, describes in *Dentistry Then and Now* how a grand mid nineteenth-century dentist handles the sale of a particular full ivory set fitted with human front teeth. It had taken his assistant, Charles, between two and three weeks to carve and was for

> an elderly and vivacious duchess who arrived . . . smartly dressed in silk and adorned with diamonds. Mr X received her graciously. When she was seated in the dental chair, he had the audacity to emphasize, in Charles's presence, that both of them had worked assiduously for two months on these very difficult dentures. After viewing the restorations from various angles, he expressed the firm belief that they were 'the cream of perfection'. He next handed her ladyship a mirror to enable her to confirm this. The verdict was: 'Well, Mr X, you have renewed my youth; they are just lovely.' . . . [Mr X] informed her that his fee was £1,000, which she joyfully paid. Later he proceeded downstairs to tell Charles (who related this incident) what he had charged and to give him £10.

Overcharging, which provided some dentists with a reputed £20,000 a year, was of course encouraged by money-snobbishness, taking the best to be the most expensive. Dr Menzies Campbell describes an incident in the surgery of a dentist called Caleb Hall of Orchard Street, London:

> A distinguished-looking stranger consulted him concerning a loosely fitting artificial denture, stating that he required a new one. On this being inserted, he expressed entire satisfaction and inquired the extent of his indebtedness. 'Five guineas,' was the reply. Thereupon, the patient's demeanour changed entirely. Removing the denture and placing it on the instrument table along with five guineas, he said: 'Thank you. I am afraid I have come to the wrong dentist. Clearly, your services are not of the standard to which I am accustomed. Meantime, I shall stick to my old denture, for which I paid seventy-two guineas.'

In 1918, not before time, there was a government inquiry into the extent of the evils of dental practice by unqualified persons. The committee found, among other things, that any person, however ignorant, could inform the public that he practised dentistry; that the public had no protection except an

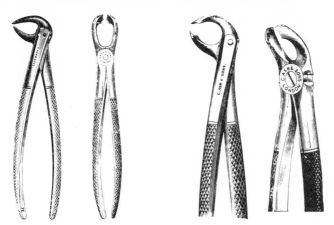

Edwardian forceps.

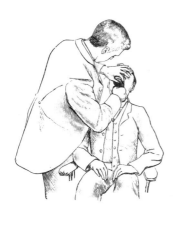

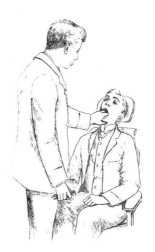

Edwardian dentist at work.

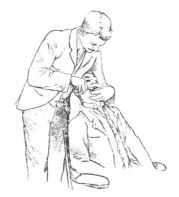

action for damages in case of injury, or the fear on the part of the operator of a possible prosecution for manslaughter in the case of a death; that the law which permitted unregistered practice produced a shortage of registered dentists because of the unattractiveness of the profession.

This alarming report at last impressed on those in authority the shortcomings of the Dentists Act of 1878. It paved the way for the more rigorous Act of 1921 which debarred all but the properly trained from carrying out dental treatment on the public.

It can at least be said that many of the unqualified men performed a useful service; they were prepared to extract teeth and fit false ones for the poor on a scale of charges within their means. However, the introduction of dental benefit on national health insurance brought better dental care within the reach of thousands previously unable to find the money.

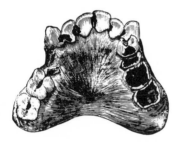
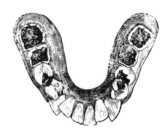

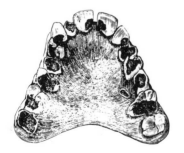

Neglected teeth of girls under 23.
From a dental book of 1900.

Dr Menzies Campbell writes thus of the typical pre-1921 quack dentist with a huge brass plate beside his door:

> An untrained woman in a nurse's uniform received callers and assured them of highly skilled attention. When a person requiring dentures had been escorted into the consulting-room, he was asked what price he was prepared to pay. Should a guinea be mentioned, the quack produced a clumsy specimen with ugly dark teeth, remarking that this was the cheapest, but there were others much better. On occasions, as high as ten guineas was paid for full upper and lower volcanite dentures, then regarded as a very good fee by many experienced qualified dentists. After the charge had been arranged, a substantial deposit was secured and an instalments card handed to the caller. No denture was ever inserted until its entire cost had been liquidated.

It was regular practice not to allow a caller to leave until some treatment had been undertaken. Extraction treatment began with a central front tooth, since the unsightly gap ensured an early return visit.

18

False Teeth in Poetry and Prose

The strikingly mechanical appearance of the early false teeth, coupled with their disappearance just before meals, made their acquisition an event that could hardly go unremarked. Wearers put up with much cheery comment and dentists had poems addressed to them. The efforts of James Gardette are celebrated in these lines which appeared in *The American Museum* of 1790:

Gardette! 'Tis thine by study to improve
The bloom of beauty and the breath of love;
To chace from ev'ry cheek distress and pain,
And bid each drooping fair one, charm again.
What tho' the glowing cheek and sparkling eye
Some faint sensations to the heart supply,·
Celia but half her wonted charms can boast –
A faded trifler, a degraded toast –
Unless the instrument of eloquence
Through iv'ry's double rows delight each sense,
And to her wond'ring lover's soul impart,
Nature's sweet sounds, attun'd by studious art.
Even tho' genious dignify the fair,
Pleasing her words, and elegant her air,
The charms of sound and sense we often slight,
Unless another sense our souls delight;
Unless Arabia's sweets assistance lend,
And ev'ry charm with added grace befriend.
Beauty, 'tis known, too oft disgusting grows,
A vapid, scentless, nay disgusting rose,

Art can no more the fading leaves adorn;
It withers on its slighted, pitied thorn.
Gardette! Advance in thy delightful art;
Promote politeness, and inform each heart,
Add (man to charm – and woman to improve) –
To beauty's bloom the balmy breath of love.

William Green, an operator for the teeth to George III, is
celebrated in a couplet in Book Four of *The Ghost* by Charles
Churchill:

> Teeth, white as ever teeth were seen,
> Delivered from the hand of Green. . . .

The American dentist John Greenwood is referred to in the
Sentimental and Literary Magazine (1797), in 'Lines written to a
lady, who had a loose tooth extracted, and fastened in again by
drilling a hole through it, and passing two ligatures, by which
it was tied to the tooth on either side'.

> Dear Madam, tell an anxious friend,
>   What terms you live on with your Tooth;
> I hope your Jars are at an end;
>   But still I wish to know the truth.
>
> 'Tis well you was alarmed in time,
>   And took the hint and look'd about;
> He and his neighbours could not chime,
>   They threaten'd shortly to fall out.
>
> An action you commenc'd for trover,
>   And Greenwood bade contention cease;
> He took him up, and bound him over,
>   And ty'd him down to keep the peace.
>
> Now let him learn to prize his lot,
>   And try to keep within his tether;
> Let each old grievance be forgot,
>   And may you both hold long together.

The satirical note is less assertive in a poem about Dubois de Chemant, the propagator of the all-porcelain denture. For one thing the author, Général Comte de Martanges, was a genuinely satisfied patient, and for another, he had been asked for a written testimonial. De Chemant put the poem in his book and also used two of the verses to embellish a frontispiece engraving of himself. In the English edition credit for the translation went to a Mr Morton.

> Teeth thirty-two, a goodly set
> This mouth of mine did whilom grace,
> Ere time with his all conquering hand
> Dismantled and laid waste the place;
> Thanks to Chemant, in better
> State and fortified it now appears,
> Than had Vauban essay'd his skill,
> Vauban the prince of Engineers.
>
> Plants of the garden or the field,
> Ye turnips white, ye carrots red,
> Yes cucumbers and olives green,
> And artichokes with towring head,
> Approach and bid the drawbridge pass
> That guards my mouth with double chain.
> Downwards with ease descend you way,
> But hope not to return again.
>
> E'en helpless infants, whilst we press
> The cradle, sprouts the pearly tooth,
> And faithful to its trust remains
> Throughout the holiday of youth.
> But years advance and teeth decay,
> Thus mystic nature has decreed.
> Then Chemant brings a second set –
> Long may he live, our friend in need!
>
> Well versed in wisdom's lore, he makes
> The *utile* and *dulce* meet,

It's his highest pitch of art
To blend the useful with the sweet.
When time has stripped our armoury bare,
Chemant steps in with subtle heed;
New grinders and new cutters gives;
With his we laugh, with his we feed.
Long live Chemant, our friend in need!

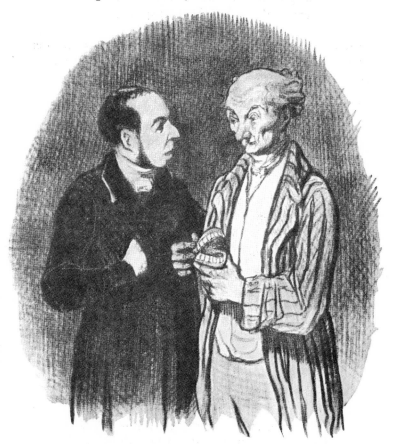

The very latest model baron. Chews by itself without ceasing.

Without ceasing! I don't want it then. One could be ruined by beef steaks with such a device.

Drawing by Honoré Daumier. Published in Charivari, *1845, as part of a series called* The Lovely Days of Life.

Ah! could so far his art extend,
Could he with teeth our youth restore;
The live-long day I'd chaunt his praise,
And as my guardian saint adore:
But ah! these joys suit not fourscore;
Backwards his flight Time will not wing,
In spite of teeth, we are proscribed
Perpetual youth, perpetual spring.

An American poem of the 1830s, written by the dentist
Solyman Brown, made a bravely optimistic claim for the dental
art of those days. Here are parts of it:

I whispered to my heart – we'll fondly seek
The means, the hour, to hear the angel speak;
For sure such language from those lips must flow,
As none but pure and seraph natures know.

'Twas said – 'twas done – the fit occasion came,
As if to quench betimes the kindling flame
Of love and admiration – for she spoke,
And lo! the heavenly spell forever broke.

For when her parted lips disclosed to view,
Those ruined arches, veiled in ebon hue . . .
Hope, disappointed, silently retired,
Disgust triumphant came, and love expired!

Let every fair one shun Urilla's fate,
And awake to action, ere it be too late; –
Let each successive day unfailing bring
The brush, the dentifrice, and, from the spring,
The cleansing flood – the labor will be small,
Or, if her past neglect preclude relief,
By gentle means like these, assuage her grief;
The dental art can remedy the ill,
Restore her hopes, and make her lovely still.

In the 1920s false teeth began to appear in British novels to suggest character and to point up scenes of embarrassment, pathos and domestic disorder. It became almost a convention that insecure or troublesome ones make a suitable attribute for

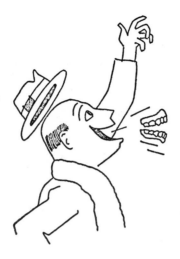

Inexperienced wearer who cheers too enthusiastically at a football match.

a person who is himself in some way insecure. In *The Forsyte Saga* Galsworthy brings in dental embarrassment to accentuate a nervous situation experienced in a tea shop by Soames Forsyte:

> At that moment, most awkward of his existence, crowded with ghosts and shadows from the past, in the presence of the only two women he had ever loved. . . . He bit too hastily at the nougat, and it stuck to his plate . . . he wiggled his finger desperately. Plate! did Jolyon wear a plate? Did that woman wear a plate?

In H. E. Bates's touching story *The Major of Hussars*, a double set of teeth, cherished and gleaming but inclined to slip, comes between an elderly man and his far-too-young wife. The story ends with an overheard bedroom scene in which the young woman hurls the teeth against a wall.

Anthony Powell created a character called Bithel, temperamentally and socially insecure, whose 'astonishingly badly fitting false teeth' make part of his performance throughout two novels, *The Valley of Bones* and *The Soldier's Art*. They seem a necessary attribute, like his furtive look, flabby hand and stained lapels. Bithel, a war-time officer, is always on the verge of trouble. On being roused after an evening of too many drinks, there, beside the bed, along with sleeping pills

> was another exhibit, something of peculiar horror. . . . Before going to sleep, Bithel had placed his false teeth in the ashtray. He had removed them bodily, the jaws still clenched on the stub of the cigar.

Bithel's brother officer, who roused him, is put in mind of an excavated tomb and of the fascination that might be aroused in archaeologists of a thousand years hence at finding the fossilized vestiges of corpse and related objects.

19

Modern False Teeth

Today it is common for people to wear such life-like false teeth that no one suspects they are not natural. Increasingly dentists take the opportunity of recording the natural teeth with impressions and photographs before they come out. By these means the colour, shape and arrangement can be copied exactly (some patients even ask for blackened teeth to be artificially reproduced). And the contours of the mouth can be kept the same by suitable building-up of the plate.

As the years go by the chin invariably gets nearer the nose and fine lines form round the mouth. These changes can be flatteringly disguised by adding bulk to existing sets of teeth, thus supporting the tissues of the face. In particular the lifting of the corners of a drooping mouth, turning a melancholy expression into a serene one, can have a strong psychological effect.

A few decades ago it was the usual procedure to allow a patient to wait for a few months without teeth while the gums healed. Apart from the inconvenience and embarrassment of going about toothless, there was sometimes the drawback of certain things happening to the mouth and face in a long waiting period which made the eventual fitting of teeth difficult. It is possible for gums to be damaged and for facial lines to appear which no dentist can remove.

Nowadays there *need* not be the least interval between having teeth out and new ones in. The dentist can make models of all the gums with the natural teeth still in place and prepare new teeth in advance. He puts them in within minutes of the old ones coming out.

It has been known for a person to make the exchange without even his own family suspecting it. He explains his refusal to eat grilled steak by remarking that he has just had a tooth out. Occasionally the teeth of actresses have changed from natural to false in the course of the shooting of a film.

It sounds painful to wear a hard set of false teeth on top of sore gums but, as explained in a helpful American booklet,[1] in practice the plates shield them from the irritation of tongue movements and food, reduce the inevitable slight bleeding and allow soothing lotions to stay where they are needed instead of being washed away. Healing is quicker, too, and those who like to bring their jaws together from time to time can of course do so without strain. Eating may not be comfortable, but it is more comfortable than with naked, uncovered gums. The only disadvantage of the immediate method is the need for numerous visits to the dentist before he undertakes the permanent sets.

Current methods of making false teeth are now almost standard. After examining the mouth, the dentist takes impressions of the upper and lower jaws and then builds casts of them by pouring plaster of Paris into the impressions. Sets of teeth could be built on these reproductions, but generally further impressions of the mouth are taken.

Almost certainly, plates made to fit the stone casts also fit the mouth perfectly. But this is not enough: the lower teeth must meet the upper ones with the jaws the right distance apart and in the right relationship to one another.

Having decided which is the proper relationship, or bite, the dentist attaches the upper and lower casts of the jaws to a machine called an articulator, which reproduces chewing motions. With the machine adjusted, temporary base plates are formed directly on the casts. Then the teeth are arranged and secured with wax: the trial dentures are ready for trying in. If the appearance is unsatisfactory, some or all of the teeth can be taken off and replaced with others which are lighter or darker or of different size or shape. This is the time for the patient to make comments. Some dentists like to have a friend of the

[1] Victor H. Sears, *New Teeth for Old*, Saint Louis, 1965.

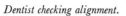

Dentist checking alignment.

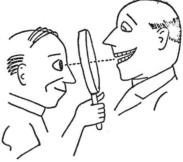

patient or a member of his family on hand to help decide on the best appearance.

When all present agree that the false teeth look well, the dentist makes sure they come together correctly, then removes them and puts them back on their casts for converting into a permanent condition.

The casts and wax trial dentures are invested in heavy metal cases constructed in sections which fit together accurately but can be taken apart during the processing. The trial dentures are embedded completely in an investment material which is poured in stage by stage.

When the investment material has hardened, the whole is warmed to soften the wax, and two halves of the container are prised apart. Then all the wax is cleaned out, leaving the teeth

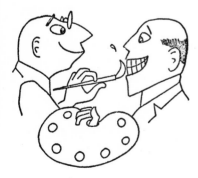

Getting the colour right.

embedded in hard investment material. Where the wax plate was, there is now a hollow space. This space is filled with one of the acrylic resins which hardens under heat and pressure to constitute the finished base, with teeth attached. All the investment material is cleaned away and the sets of teeth brushed and polished ready for final adjustment in the patient's mouth.

For the front teeth, the material used is usually porcelain or acrylic resin. Porcelain was almost the only material used until a few years ago, before the plastics were introduced. Plastic teeth are not ideal, though with their lifelike colouring and translucency they are certainly better than the cheaper porcelain ones. Moreover they stick to the acrylic resin bases so tightly as to form almost one single piece of material.

The back teeth, which take the wear and tear of chewing, may also be made of either porcelain or plastics. The disadvantage of porcelain back teeth is that when they come together they make a sharp clicking sound. Plastics, being softer, do not: but they wear down faster. Some dentists have tried putting porcelain teeth on one plate and plastic on the other – only to find that though noise is reduced, wear on the plastic teeth is greatly increased.

The chewing surfaces of the back teeth are made in different designs. It might be thought that artificial teeth that perfectly resembled the natural ones would be best for chewing. In practice the reproduced projections, or cusps, of natural teeth can easily unseat a denture. Sliding on the gums not only causes unsatisfactory chewing but may gradually destroy the all-important ridges. Back teeth that are fairly flat have been found to work best.

As he goes through the various steps in making a set of false teeth the dentist of today has the following objectives always in mind: that the teeth should be pleasant and appropriate to look at, comfortable and firm; that they should allow clear speech, chew well, hold the jaws the proper distance apart and restore natural contours to the lips and cheeks; that their design should be such as to protect the supporting gum and bone.

Making false teeth stay in place can still be a problem. With

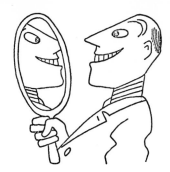

Satisfied wearer.

certain mouths even the most carefully made sets cannot be made more than tolerably secure. Cushions and pads applied by patients sometimes make matters worse by causing the teeth to come together the wrong way. For some years the use of opposing magnets built into the upper and lower plates was considered the ideal solution: like the old coil springs, the magnets exerted pressure to force the two sets away from one another. Unfortunately they worked best when least needed – that is, the nearer the sets of teeth were together. As the mouth is opened wide, in laughing, for example, so the magnetic force grows less, until, with the jaws at full stretch, it ceases to operate at all.

About fifteen years ago successful experiments were carried out in America and other countries with the so-called implant method of securing full dentures. By this method metal plates are screwed or otherwise attached to the bone of the jaw, leaving metal posts projecting through the gum. False teeth fitted on these are as immovable as fixed bridgework. A highly skilled surgical operation is necessary of course, but this exotic form of treatment can at least be borne in mind as a last resort by people growing tired of the nuisance of a floating lower set.

20

Identification by False Teeth

The characteristics of the teeth, especially their fillings or inlays, have often helped to identify dead bodies. False teeth can be of peculiar usefulness: some dentist is likely to have kept a model, or at least a record, of the jaws they were made for. False teeth will survive intense heat, even erosion by acid, without losing individual detail. Lawrence's Arab found crushing his false teeth to bits with a large stone[1] – as a penance for eating infidel food – probably left fragments in the sand that would have been recognizable to his dentist.

Thus even if a body has been deliberately mutilated, or is reduced to a heap of bones, the police can expect to identify it if any sort of denture is present.

The importance of false teeth in forensic work was first fully realized in the extraordinary Parkman case in America.[2] Dr George Parkman, a respected figure at Harvard University, failed to return home for dinner on 23 November 1849. He was sixty-four and a man of regular habits. He had simply disappeared.

Suspicion at length fell on his colleague John White Webster, professor of chemistry at the University; he had been behaving furtively, and it was known that he owed Parkman money. Webster's chemical laboratory was searched. In a tea chest were found various human remains and, in the ashes of an assay furnace, small fragments of a lower jaw bone, three blocks of artificial teeth in porcelain and some melted gold.

[1] T. E. Lawrence, *The Seven Pillars of Wisdom*, 1935.
[2] G. Dilnot, *The Trial of Professor Webster, Famous Trials Series*, 1928.

At Webster's trial for murder a dentist called Nathan Keep identified the teeth as parts of an upper and lower denture he had made for Parkman three years earlier. He clearly remembered all the circumstances.

Dr Parkman, he said, had been anxious about the teeth being ready in time for the opening of a new medical college at which he might have to give a speech. The work progressed smoothly till the day before the event, when some of the bottom teeth collapsed in a baking process. He and his assistant worked on the dentures all night, but even so they were fitted in Dr Parkman's mouth, with gold coil springs, only thirty minutes before the ceremony.

Dr Parkman returned shortly afterwards complaining that the lower set cramped his tongue. Rather reluctantly, because it spoiled the finish, Keep ground away parts of the inner surface. Dr Parkman's last visit to him had been a fortnight before his disappearance. He had called late at night for an urgent repair following the breakage of one of the coil springs.

Keep was able to demonstrate to the court that the pieces found in the furnace fitted the plaster model of Parkman's jaw which was in his possession. He drew attention to marks made by the grinding operation he had carried out.

In answer to a question from the defence, why the teeth had not perished in the heat, Keep explained that if they had been left in the mouth the cranium would have acted as a muffle. The dental evidence was unassailable. Webster was found guilty and hanged.

False teeth provided damning evidence in the Acid Bath case of 1949.[1] Mrs Durand-Deacon, a rich widow living at the Onslow Court Hotel, South Kensington, went out one afternoon in February in the company of a man called John Haigh, who was also a resident at the hotel. She never reappeared. Next day Haig escorted a friend of hers to Chelsea Police Station to report the disappearance. A woman police officer felt

---

[1] Keith Simpson, *British Dental Journal*, 6 November 1951. *The Dentist's Handbook on Law and Ethics*, 1962.

suspicious about Haig; she did not like the look of him. It was found that he had a record of forgery and theft.

Inquiries were made at business premises of Haigh's at Crawley in Sussex – a two-floor shed used for what he called experiments. Some strange things were discovered: carboys of sulphuric acid, papers relating to the death of five other people who had disappeared without trace, a pistol and, on a wall, tiny blood stains of the kind that would be made if a person standing there was shot through the head.

At his fourth interview with the police, Haigh became boastful, as criminals often do, and admitted having killed Mrs Durand-Deacon and destroyed her body in acid. 'But every trace has gone,' he said. 'How can you prove murder if there is no body?' It was a preposterous challenge, leading to an intense search.

On the ground outside the shed lay a mass of black sludge. Careful sifting of this brought to light three human gall stones, part of a left foot and some eroded fragments of human bone showing signs of arthritis. But there was nothing that could be said to be the remains of Mrs Durand-Deacon; nothing that would enable the Crown pathologist to say more than that the remains were human and those of a female who was probably elderly.

On the third day of debris-sifting, however, there appeared first an upper, then a lower set of false teeth. They had almost entirely resisted the action of the acid.

Miss Helen Mayo, Mrs Durand-Deacon's dentist, was able to identify the teeth. She could say at Lewes Assizes: 'That is my work. I made them for Mrs Durand-Deacon.' Miss Mayo demonstrated that they fitted the models she had made of her patient's mouth two years earlier and pointed out alterations she had made. As Mrs Durand-Deacon had been fussy about her appearance, indeed a rather exacting patient, the plates had on several occasions been built up. Miss Mayo said she could describe the sets of teeth from her notes without seeing them. Her unshakeable evidence led to Haigh being found guilty of the murder of Mrs Durand-Deacon.

As the teeth were made of acrylic resin, which is only temporarily resistant to acid, it was fortunate that Haigh made his statement when he did and that the teeth were found not more than a fortnight after the old lady's disappearance: experiments have shown that a lump of acrylic resin put in strong sulphuric acid will dissolve completely in about three weeks.

A few years ago the badly disintegrated remains of a woman were found in Epping Forest. There were no papers that would identify the body; but there was a denture, a three-tooth piece lying underneath the head. It neatly fitted the upper jaw although most of the teeth had fallen away. A dentist produced records which corresponded perfectly and thereby established identity.

In the Carron murder case in Australia the victim's body was thoroughly burned, but several artificial teeth of a type known as diatoric came to light among the ashes. A dentist was able to say that in making the person believed killed a denture, he had used this type of tooth in its construction.

On 17 September 1949, the lives of 118 people were lost in an appalling fire on the S.S. *Noronic* while she was in Toronto harbour. The evidence of false teeth, carefully tabulated, proved of great usefulness in putting names to bodies made unrecognizable by the flames.

The procedure is not always so straightforward. To actually prove a corpse's identity by means of false teeth is only possible when teeth have some distinctive feature and when the appropriate model of the jaws can be produced. In 1942 the police of New Rochelle photographed a set of teeth found on a body and had it published in a dental journal; they also exhibited the teeth themselves at a dental convention attended by over 10,000 dentists. Despite the publicity, they remained unrecognized.

Index of Persons